Some Reader Responses to *Dancing with the Rhythms of Life*

"Dancing with the Rhythms of Life is so easy to read. The conversational style really pulls you in, and the advice is a natural part of the conversation. The examples and stories make it real and relatable. The result is that readers are treated as if they have intelligence, instead as (as often happens) as if ordinary people just can't understand. Dr. Rothschild leaps over this and makes it clear that you can. This is a great gift, especially when our health is front-and-center."

—MADELYN BLAIR, PH.D., author,
Unlocked: Discover How to Embrace the Unexpected

"Dr. Rothschild's book reads just as she practices medicine, reflecting her wise intuition and talented diagnostic skills. Easy to read, this book shares stories of how patients are helped to resolve their health issues, searching for the root cause that may include more than just a physiological rationale. How refreshing in this day and age!"

—HEATHER WURZER, Certified Holistic Health Coach

"Dancing with the Rhythms of Life is a guide for those who want a partner along their path to wellness. Dr. Rothschild reveals that Listening is the key to health. This book encourages—actually teaches—readers how to partner with a healthcare professional to be able to dance with the Rhythms of Life from birth to death."

—Jo ISRAELSON, MFA, educator, community-based artist,
www.thestonepath.wordpress.com

D1546428

DANCING WITH THE RHYTHMS OF LIFE

A HOLISTIC DOCTOR'S GUIDE FOR WOMEN

~

Marianne Rothschild, M.D.

— GAIA HEALING —

Gaia Healing
www.dancingwiththerhythmsoflife.com

Disclaimer: *Dancing with the Rhythms of Life* is intended solely for information and educational purposes and not as personal medical advice. Please consult your health care professional if you have any questions about your health.

Editor & Publishing Coordinator: Naomi Rose, *www.naomirose.net*

Cover Illustration: Lucyann Foronda Dirksen, *www.lfdstudios.com*

Book Design & Typesetting: Margaret Copeland/Terragrafix, *www.terragrafix.com*

Dancing with the Rhythms of Life: A Holistic Doctor's Guide for Women /
Marianne Rothschild, M.D.

First edition. Published 2020.

Printed in the United States of America.

ISBN #: 978-1-7349349-0-8

This book is dedicated to the generations to come with the hope that we leave them the gifts of love and respect for our most wonderful and dear planet Earth and an understanding of the reciprocity of all Life.

Acknowledgments

This book would not have been possible without the help of many people.

I especially want to thank my brother, Peter Graumann, for his tireless encouragement, humor, and support through the whole process.

A thousand thank-yous to Naomi Rose, my book midwife, and Max Regan, my writing coach. Their skill, advice, expertise, and guidance were invaluable.

Great gratitude to Pat Chicon, Liz Rothschild, Adam Twine, Curtis Ewing, Heather Wurzer, Jo Israelson, Madelyn Blair, and Randy Mack for their feedback and caring encouragement.

Deep bow to my dear friend Jenaii Gold for her ongoing companionship and insight throughout the journey.

Much love and gratitude to my daughter Molly McMahon for her knowledgeable contributions and skillful proofreading; my son, Peter Doshi, for editing and insights; and my daughter Verushka Doshi for her unflagging enthusiasm and timely pep talks.

To Sally Fallon Morell for her knowledgeable support and encouragement.

To my dear Shawn Connors for graciously typing and rewriting endlessly and cheerfully.

And to all my family and great circle of friends, as well as my wonderful patients who cheered me on and gave me confidence that my efforts were worthwhile—you are the wind beneath my wings. Bless you all.

Deep bow to all who have inspired me, taught me, and from whose lives and work I have been nourished: Dr. Bill Mebane; Ebun Laughing Crow Adelona, Ph.D.; Atul Gawande, M.D.; Guru Maharaji; Dr. Albert Schweitzer; James Hollis, Ph.D.; Martin Prechtel; Pema Chodron; Alan Gaby, M.D; Dr. William Crook; and Dr. John Lee.

Table of Contents

~

MY PERSONAL JOURNEY IN
HOLISTIC MEDICINE

I took my good health for granted as a child and rarely saw a doctor. I had the usual childhood illnesses of my time—measles, chicken pox, German measles—and recovered uneventfully from them. My first major encounter with conventional allopathic medical care came in my early twenties.

As a young inexperienced first-time mother, I became impatient after several days of dealing with a snotty-nosed and cranky toddler, so I took her to a doctor. I left with an antibiotic. The next morning, I woke to find that my child had turned into a pumpkin. Her face was swollen and there was a bright red rash all over her body. I was shocked and frightened. I never suspected that allopathic medicine could be harmful or dangerous. Her unfortunate adverse reaction prompted me to research safer options that I could use to help her get well. Over the years, I continue to learn.

I learned that my toddler's cold was caused by a virus. I learned that antibiotics do not destroy viruses. I learned about particular herbs and homeopathic medicines that help fight viruses, and about the power of Vitamin C to boost the immune system and reduce infections. Over time, my knowledge and confidence in these alternative methods grew as I used them on myself, my child, my friends, and the rest of my family. Not only were these alternatives effective, but they also were safe. There was no risk of harm.

My life reached a turning point during the 1970s. I was living and working as a lay midwife, serving the homebirth community in rural California. The homebirth movement was growing, largely fed by families who wished to avoid the many mandatory interventions commonly practiced in hospital deliveries. Being a midwife brought together my knowledge and skill in natural healing techniques, my joy at being part of people's intimate life experiences, and my desire to be of service to others. At that time, lay midwives were unable to obtain legal or licensed status in

California. Perhaps if fate had not intervened, I might still be that mid-wife.

Everything changed for me when I attended a home birth and, unfortunately, the baby was stillborn. Unexpectedly, I was arrested a few weeks later and spent a day in jail. It was a frightening experience and I felt at great peril. If convicted, I could have gone to prison for up to twenty years. At that time, midwifery, which has a history as old as time, was in question in California. Although the charges against me were eventually dismissed, it was clear that I could not continue to practice as a lay midwife and put myself and my family in further jeopardy. This was a powerful turning point in my life.

I looked at various career paths and ultimately chose medicine. Life as a medical doctor seemed to offer me the greatest flexibility of application and the most credibility—or, put more simply, maximum freedom and power. During my seven years of pre-med, medical school, and residency, I told very few people of my interest in holistic alternatives or my midwifery experiences. I felt like a sheep in wolf's clothing.

After completing a three-year residency in Family Practice, I was overjoyed to join a holistic family practice. It was a friendly, collaborative, and stimulating atmosphere. We four doctors shared one large office room and would frequently "curbside consult" each other on difficult patients. One doctor practiced acupuncture, another homeopathy, and the nurse practitioner was an experienced herbalist. My skills and experience in holistic medicine grew logarithmically.

Later, I moved to Maryland and joined a primary-care practice run by Johns Hopkins Medical Services Corporation. But after three and a half years of seeing a patient every fifteen minutes, I was frustrated, burned out, and ready for a change. Serendipity and a leap of faith brought me to establish a solo holistic medical practice in my home office, and I have been practicing there happily ever since.

By the time my patients are sitting with me in my office, they have already traveled down winding country roads through vistas of gently rolling hills and walked the fifty yards of gravel pathway through the garden to my office door. Many have told me how much they enjoy the experience of coming to my office. I am convinced that Mother Nature does a good deal of the healing before I ever even see them.

Then we sit together. I ask them to tell me why they have come. And I am quiet and listen. I listen until they are complete. Some people have never been able to tell their whole story. After years of listening to patients tell their stories, I have learned that if I listen long enough and carefully enough, people will not only tell me what is going on but also what they need to get better.

My listening is holistic, multifaceted. Peoples' lives are like tapestries, woven with many threads. I take in their stories, the feeling tones, their physical presence, and their past and current life situation. Together we look at the laboratory and other test data they have brought, their food journal, and any prescriptions or nutritional supplements they are taking. We often sit for several hours. Sometimes a certain alchemy of healing occurs when I sit together with my patient that no book can reproduce.

At the end of our session, I provide my feedback regarding what I think may be going on and what approaches might be helpful. Then together, we decide what we are going to work on and our next steps. I tell my patient that we are now a team, and I commit to be part of their support network as we go forward.

PART ONE

~

THE CORE RHYTHMS

Building a Strong Foundation of Health

Introduction

"The expert at anything was once a beginner." —HELEN HAYES

Women know something about the rhythms of life. Growing up they experience distinct life cycles and stages. Each of these brings with it physical, mental and emotional changes that can challenge a woman's health and wellbeing. When we learn to recognize and dance with these rhythms in our life, we experience less stress and more joy.

Over many years as a holistic physician sharing my patients' stories and health concerns, I uncovered the Five Essential Rhythms of Health. These Essential Rhythms compose the foundation necessary to build the vitality of the body, mind and spirit—a foundation strong enough to withstand the vicissitudes of time and disease. I have shared these foundational Rhythms with many patients and I have seen their health improve and their lives become more joyful as they learned to dance with these Rhythms.

PART ONE of *Dancing with the Rhythms of Life* reveals the specific elements needed to build a strong foundation of health. Each chapter focuses on one of the five foundational pillars. In Chapter One you will learn what it means to live in harmony with Life's Universal Rhythms. The steps to attain and maintain the rhythm of good digestion are explained in Chapter Two. Chapter Three contains detailed information on what comprises a balanced rhythm of optimal nourishment. And in Chapter Four you will receive guidance on vitalizing movement and how to include it in your life. Chapter Five explores the rhythm of emotional wellbeing and offers holistic treatments.

Our lives flow more smoothly when these realms function well. Once we fully appreciate the importance of these rhythms and understand how to work with them, we can choose to flow with the river of life rather than push against the flow. The Five Core Rhythms are key to creating and maintaining health.

Real health means *extraordinary living*. This is not just a matter of choosing the "right" foods or digesting "well," nor is it about getting the "right" exercise or achieving the "right" emotional state.

The purpose of this book is not to provide another "cookbook" with an exact program to "fix" yourself or your health problems. For one thing, everyone is unique, so there is no one-size-fits-all "cure." For another, there are too many "self help" books out there already—each with their implied message that "something is wrong with you."

What I hope to provide is awareness and education about the expansiveness of "normal," and a holistic perspective of what comprises "good living." Holistic medicine invites us to step back and get a broader and deeper perspective on what is really going on.

When patients first come to see me, they have already made a decision to *do something* about their health. When you picked up this book—whether out of vague curiosity or a specific desire for greater health—you have already taken the first step on your own healing journey. Welcome!

CHAPTER ONE

SYNCHRONY

Dancing with the Universal Rhythms of Life

"The Earth does not belong to man; Man belongs to the Earth. This we know. All things are connected like the blood which unites one family. Whatever befalls the Earth befalls the sons of the Earth. Man did not weave the web of life, he is merely a strand in it. Whatever he does to the web, he does to himself." —CHIEF SEATTLE

Truly extraordinary living involves holding an awareness of the universal rhythms and cycles of life, and moving in harmony with them. *Life has Rhythms!* These rhythms already exist in our world, in our universe—and in our bodies. When we honor them and live in accord with these rhythms, cycles, and principles of Life, we experience greater ease and flow. These rhythms are impersonal and universal, and at the same time intimate and very personally experienced. To the extent that we are aware of them, we understand the nature of our cells, tissues, and life itself. These rhythms form an orderly system that has always existed. When we recognize and appreciate them, we are able to "go with the flow" rather than "against the grain."

Some say we humans have lost our "Original Instructions." Animals, insects, and plants appear to have been born knowing *their* "Original Instructions." They know how to find food, water, and shelter. They don't need a class to teach them how to nurture their young, or when to prepare for winter, or how and where to build their homes. They seem to have found a way to synchronize with the Rhythms of Nature. And they flourish when they are in harmony with them.

Like them, we also can flourish, once we understand and honor these "Original Instructions" by dancing with the Rhythms of Life.

The Rhythm of the Day

Who hasn't heard the old saying, "Early to bed, early to rise makes a man healthy, wealthy, and wise"? The question is: do we *live* by its wisdom? We are all familiar with the rhythm of the day—punctuated by sunrise at daybreak; midday, with the sun at its highest point; and nighttime, once the sun has left the sky.

If we have had sufficient rest (human beings, by and large, are not nocturnal creatures), we wake up in the morning with energy for our day. If we are lucky, we might even wake up early enough to be greeted by the dawn chorus, courtesy of our feathered songbird friends. If we are busy and active during the day, by late afternoon our energy is waning, and once it is night we do best to head for bed.

Synchronizing with the rhythm of the day provides us with maximum energy when we need it and a restful sleep at night. People whose jobs require that they work at night often have difficulties—not only with sleep, but also with other health issues, as a result of living out of sync with the Rhythm of the Day. People whose work involves constantly changing shifts (such as firemen, policemen, and nurses) suffer even more. They never have time to establish a rhythm at all. Their schedules are constantly in flux, and eventually their health decompensates.

> *Synchronizing with the Rhythm of the Day provides us with maximum energy when we need it and a restful sleep at night.*

I have seen many people improve their health and sense of wellbeing by bringing their activities into closer harmony with the Rhythm of the day.

THE RHYTHMS OF THE SEASONS

Not only does the day have rhythms that serve us when we align with them, but so do the *seasons*. We can become aware of these seasonal rhythms by observing them in the natural world around us. Each of the four seasons brings a particular energy, a particular focus and mood. Through understanding the nature of each season, we can learn a lot about right timing for our own wellbeing.

Spring's rhythm has a push in it. Like new shoots on a plant, it thrusts upward and out. After a winter rest, life energy wants to move. Intuitively, we already know this energy. It feels revitalizing. We talk about having a "spring" in our step, and of new ideas "springing" into our heads.

Summer's rhythm is a full-tilt boogie. With long days and short nights, we are dancing hard. The sun is at its zenith for the year, and all of nature is bus-tling. Brooks are babbling, plants are making fruit and seed, bees are buzzing, and animals are tending their young. Everything in nature is active and busy ensuring life's continuation.

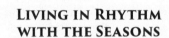

LIVING IN RHYTHM WITH THE SEASONS

Spring — new beginnings
Summer — maximum activity
Autumn — harvest time and letting go
Winter — deep rest and quiet

The *Autumn* rhythm is slower and more deliberate. This is a time of harvest, when nature prepares for the coming winter. Some creatures migrate to other lands, while others get ready to hibernate or become dormant. The trees let go of their leaves and call their sap back into the ground, where it can be stored safe from harm. Some creatures will gestate their young over the winter and give birth in the Spring. We see how, in Autumn, nature organizes and lays down the blue-print for the coming year with seeds designed to remain dormant until the up-thrusting energy of Spring wakens them.

Winter's rhythm is one of deep rest and quiet. The days are short and the nights are long. This is a time to hunker down. Activity is limited to what is absolutely necessary to maintain life. Stillness prevails. Without the deep restorative rest of Winter, there will be no energy to burst forth in the spring.

How Do the Rhythms of the Seasons Manifest in Our Lives?

Our life is a garden, and we can become skillful gardeners, connecting the Rhythm of the Seasons with the undertakings in our life. There is a Springtime, when new growth appears. Care needs to be taken to shelter the new "plants" from harm and weed out what may jeopardize them. Summer is a season when garden activity is at a peak and we are busy tending many projects. The day is never long enough to complete all that is wanting to be done. In the Fall, we harvest what we have grown. We sort through our garden and let go of what is no longer needed. And in the Winter, the garden rests and is quiet.

We can use the principles of gardening through the four seasons to bring balance into our lives. Do we allow space for new things to sprout up? Are we always going full-speed as if it is always Summer? Do we take time to evaluate what is no longer needed and let it go? Are we giving ourselves a time for real rest? *To acknowledge a life that has seasons is to restore harmony and dance with Life's Rhythms.*

By observing these rhythms in nature, we learn that there is a time when it is appropriate to push forward; a time to inaugurate new plans; and an equally appropriate time to pull in—to gestate, to consolidate, and to rest. The rhythms in nature are expansion and contraction, activity and stillness, growth and decay. Life occurs in rhythms of cycles and seasons.

When we honor these natural rhythms as they manifest in ourselves, we wait for inspiration to arise in its right time rather than forcing it; we acknowledge the need for rest after activity; we feed our hungers; and we dance our joy. When we value the principle of right timing, we synchronize with the natural rhythms, and our energy is dynamic and sustainable.

As a culture, however, we tend to ignore the lessons we could learn from the Rhythms of the Seasons. We no longer validate the rhythmic need for rest by observing a Sabbath day. Instead, we push on without a day of rest. Today, few businesses close on Sundays or holidays, and some stay open twenty-four hours a day. We ignore the seasonal hint of the Winter darkness telling us to slow down. Instead, we force ourselves into even *more* activity during the Winter holiday season. Many times, we reap the bitter harvest of failing to harmonize with these rhythms, and suffer increased stress, fatigue, illness, anxiety, and depression.

When we honor these natural rhythms as they manifest in ourselves, we wait for inspiration to arise in its right time rather than forcing it; we acknowledge the need for rest after activity; we feed our hungers; and we dance our joy. When we value the principle of right timing, we synchronize with the natural rhythms, and our energy is dynamic and sustainable.

Integrating Nature's Rhythm of the Seasons into Your Life

You don't have to continue being at the effect of a non-rhythmic way of life. You can *choose* to harmonize with the seasonal energies. Take more rest in the Winter, and plan your greatest activity for Summer. Join in the generative energy of the Springtime with new plans and projects, and sort through your harvest in the Fall, keeping only what is still valuable.

We live in a culture that doesn't value these rhythms. We are bombarded with messages to be more productive, more efficient, more this and more that. The presence of coffee shops on every corner urges us to drink more coffee so that we *never* need to stop. Or better yet, have a New-Age energy drink, which will keep you hopping along even longer.

The word *convalescence*—once a perfectly acceptable description of the time it takes to renew a depleted body, mind, or spirit—has disappeared from common use. Words like *respite, delay,* and *retreat* have become synonyms for defeat and failure, rather than judicious choices for maintaining balance and health. (As in: "I'm going to *delay* my meeting until I've had a chance to rest and recharge." "I need a *respite* from so much productivity." "A *retreat* will clarify and restore me.")

In nature, we can see that life moves in cycles: of night and day, rest and activity, inspiration and expiration, growth and decay. Periods of extreme activity must be balanced with ones of deep rest. This cyclic rhythm allows for rebalance and sustainability. It is self-renewing and vital.

The Rhythm of the Moon Cycle

My teacher, Laughing Crow, first introduced me to the power and benefit of working with the moon cycle. In addition to providing beauty and light, the moon has many other influences over activities here on earth. Most people are aware that the moon's gravitational pull causes the tides in the oceans. But you may not be aware that the *land* also experiences tides, and has been measured to move as much as four inches from high to low tide.

> **Harmonizing with the Rhythms of the Moon**
>
> *New (dark) moon* — new beginnings; time to make new plans, initiate a change
>
> *Full moon* — a good time to release things (material and otherwise)

Since we live within a world that is constantly experiencing the push and pull of the moon, we can assume that we also are influenced. In which case, why not *synchronize* with these rhythms?

Every 28 days, the moon travels from new moon to full moon, and back again. Farmers have long used the phases of the moon to dictate the best planting times for various crops. We can do the same with the garden of our life. When we choose our activity to coincide with the phase of the moon, we can experience greater ease in accomplishment.

- The energy of the **new** moon (also called the *dark* moon) is that of *new beginnings*. Use the new-moon time to make a new plan or to inaugurate a change.

- When the moon is **full**, things are in their *least stable state*. Emergency rooms are well aware of increased activity during the time of a full moon. Minds can become less stable, which is how the terms "lunacy" and "lunatic" got their names. Babies are more likely to be born around the full moon. You can synchronize and utilize the full-moon energy. For example, choose that time to clean out a closet or let go of something you want to release.

If you don't live where you can observe the moon directly, you can follow its changes with a lunar calendar. (The Lunar Press is an excellent resource. See notes for Chapter One in the Appendix.) A lunar year contains 13 months of 28 days each. Not only does the Lunar Press calendar provide in-depth information and interpretation about the phases of the moon, but it also graphically displays each cycle as a spiral rather than as the typical rectangular and linear format we are accustomed to seeing with calendars based on the solar 12 months.

Cycling our lives with the moon's changing influence creates synergy in our lives. Every 28 days, the moon cycles through the 12 signs of the zodiac. An awareness of where the moon is on a given day can help you align your own needs and wishes with the moon cycle to good effect. For example, when I am looking for a good day to begin a new project, I will choose a day when the moon passes through Capricorn or Aries. *Capricorn* is a good time for setting and achieving goals. Moon transiting *Aries* promotes self-expression and the initiation of new ventures. When picking a date for an important meeting, I will try to arrange it when the moon transits *Libra*, which is oriented toward co-operation and increased social interaction. (These insights come from the Lunar Calendar.)

THE RHYTHM OF CREATION AND DESTRUCTION

Another of nature's great rhythms that I have learned to identify and trust is the Rhythm of Creation and Destruction. The Rhythm of Creation includes inception, gestation, labor, and ultimately birth. The Rhythm of Destruction includes deterioration and dissolution, and, ultimately death. All creation contains within it the seeds of its death and destruction.

Labor and Birth

I learned a lot about the Rhythm of Creation by observing the stages of birthing as a midwife. Let me share some basics of the literal birthing process with you, and then fan these out and apply them to how we can use them in our lives.

Labor involves moments of extreme effort coupled with periods of rest. As I got to observe, some labors proceed slowly and steadily, while others go so rapidly that the mother-to-be can barely hang on and keep up. Still other labors come to a complete stop midway, giving opportunity for a temporary rest to the laboring mother (as well as the rest of her team) in order to be ready for the hard work that lies ahead. Each birthing journey I observed was unique and perfect in its nature and timing, and yet they all contained the same recognizable rhythm.

Labor involves moments of extreme effort coupled with periods of rest.

When we "labor" with a project, whether cleaning a room or planning a trip, the Rhythm of Labor is a reminder that there are times when great effort is required, and also times to rest—when nothing needs to be done. The pacing and duration of our undertakings will be unique, just as each woman's labor is unique, because we are each a unique being.

The Transition Stage in the Rhythm of Creation—the Pivotal Point

Transition is the time in labor when the woman's cervix is almost fully dilated. This occurs just before the urge to push appears. (Once the pushing begins, the whole tone of labor shifts into very focused birthing energy.) Almost invariably, transition is a time when labor is most intense and the laboring mother's deepest fears and doubts creep in. I remember so clearly, in my own labors, reaching a point when the contractions were so strong that I doubted I could breathe through another one. I was sure that I could not survive the intensity any longer; that I would die. I felt frightened and overwhelmed.

Fortunately, I had seasoned midwives with me. They reached out to me in that moment with words and loving touch, reassuring me that my fears were all signs that the end of labor was not far off. They reminded me that I was in Transition and that I was in the process of giving birth. I had lost sight of the reality that this intense experience was finite, and that there was a baby waiting at the end. I needed to be reassured that the journey had an end—and that the end was not my death but the birth of a new life.

A good midwife reassures the woman in labor that the fear and intensity of Transition signify the nearness of the end of the ordeal. She understands that the journey of birth is transformational, and that to transform we have to deeply let go and step through our fear in order to allow change to happen.

*Almost invariably, Transition is a time when
labor is most intense and one's deepest fears and
doubts creep in. But to transform we have to
deeply let go and step through our fear in order to
allow change to happen.*

Life is full of transitions and transformations. Sometimes we find ourselves in the midst of a difficult time in our life. We feel stuck and filled
with fear. Perhaps we might experience this period differently if we could
be aware that we are in the *Transition* stage. What if we could really see
ourselves in the midst of something new being created? It is helpful to seek
support and encouragement (whether from books or people in our lives) to
remind us that change is happening, even though we cannot see it yet.

If we can realize that we are in Transition when things feel overwhelming and scary, then we can choose to stay conscious with the pain
of our experience, rather than avoiding our fears by drugging or numbing
them. We can bring ourselves fully present to each sensation as we experience it. It takes courage to consciously breathe through the intensity, one
moment at a time.

It is difficult to remember, in the midst of those deepest, darkest
moments of extreme fear and self-doubt, that those same fears and doubts
are actually the heralds signifying that we are almost out of the woods.
Our "Transition stage" is almost over, and we are near the end of the
ordeal. If we are fortunate, we will have found some wise, midwifely voices
to provide us with reassurance and to remind us that this time won't last
forever.

*Those same fears and doubts are actually the
heralds signifying that we are almost out of the
woods. Our "Transition stage" is almost over, and
we are near the end of the ordeal.*

Take care to stay present when in Transition—don't numb out! In the
birthing process, pain medication can mask or numb the experience of the

Transition stage. If a woman is given pain medication just when the fear and overwhelm are the greatest, she will not experience how the energy shifts at the end of Transition, when the pain spontaneously disappears or resolves into the overwhelming urge to push. She may not receive the powerful confirmation of her own resiliency that enduring the pains of labor can give. Medication may diminish her sense of accomplishment or achievement. She may later judge herself as weak and inadequate to the challenge of birth.

Sometimes we find ourselves in a very painful time—a loss, a betrayal, a disappointment or stuckness—in which life feels grim, and obstacles loom seemingly too large to surmount. It is tempting to numb out with drugs or alcohol. Yet if we are numbed, we may miss the journey while in the "slough of despair." There is something to be gained from staying present in the face of fear and overwhelm.

> *There is something to be gained from staying*
> *present in the face of fear and overwhelm.*

I also know that *pain relief* in labor can be appropriate in certain circumstances. During actual labor, I have seen it be helpful and provide a temporary respite that enabled a woman to take a break and then return to her birthing, reinvigorated. We can choose pain relief not out of the fear that we cannot survive, but rather to provide us with a further tool to navigate through our labor. The presence of a knowledgeable guide through our birthing journey can be a vital source of support. Depending on what we are birthing, that guide could be a doula or midwife, or a mentor appropriate to what is being birthed or created.

When life feels grim and painful, we can find temporary relief by watching a funny movie, spending time with friends, getting a massage, or taking a trip. These activities can provide a welcome and needed break and allow us to return to our situation reinvigorated.

The Rhythm of Dissolution and Death

Sometimes we are least prepared for the *second* part of the Rhythm of Creation—Death and Destruction. We have a hard time letting go of old circumstances and connections. Despite all the evidence that change is inevitable, we often refuse to accept it. We steadfastly maintain our belief that everything will always stay the same.

It is most helpful to learn to graciously bend with the changes so that we are not broken; to accept that loss is an intrinsic part of life. Many helpful books are available to ease the grief and pain that often come with loss. I recommend Pema Chodron's *When Things Fall Apart* and James Hollis' *Swamplands of the Soul: New Life in Dismal Places.*

> *It is most helpful to learn to graciously bend with the changes so that we are not broken; to accept that loss is an intrinsic part of life.*

THE RHYTHM OF RECIPROCITY AND GENEROSITY

Living in harmony with the universal Rhythm of Reciprocity and Generosity means acknowledging that everything we do has an impact. In physics, we have the law that "every action has an equal and opposite reaction." Another law of physics states: "Energy can be neither created nor destroyed." If we *take*, we must *give back* to rebalance. Energetically, this means that there is no "free lunch." When we fail to acknowledge this universal principle of reciprocity, our life becomes imbalanced and unsustainable.

Each of us was *given* life. We didn't buy our life or do anything to deserve it—it is a gift. We teach our children to say "thank you" when they are given a gift. How do we give thanks for this gift of life we have been given? Much of the time, we are so lost in the details of our life that we lose sight of the big picture—that *this life itself is a gift.* Doing things that acknowledge the gift opens the heart and brings a sense of joy. Gratitude is an experience of acknowledgment for a gift that has been given. It is part of the Rhythm of Reciprocity.

Sometimes when I sit with someone who has serious health concerns, I ask them "And when you are well again, what will you do with the gift of health you've been given? Is there something that you want to contribute, in the spirit of reciprocity, to express your gratitude?" Having a vision or goal beyond just "feeling better" opens us to greater possibilities when it is difficult to see the way ahead.

Our lives and our health are intrinsically linked with the web of life of this planet and all life on it. When we share with others (our time, focus, energy, money, life force) because we are called to do so without expecting a return, we contribute to the health and wellbeing of all, including ourselves. This is a truth that we can learn from the honeybees. Their simple daily work benefits the health of not only the whole hive but also the whole earth.

Most of humankind has long forgotten to apply the Rhythm of Reciprocity to our relationship with the earth. We suck out the oil, we drain the swamps to develop the land, we destroy the rainforest, we pollute the waters. We use and abuse. We do not return things as we found them. We do not plan to restore what we have taken. We ignore this Universal Rhythm of Reciprocity—and we are reaping the consequences on the physical, emotional, and spiritual levels.

Ancient people around the world were well aware of this Rhythm of Reciprocity. They held ceremonies and made prayers before going out to hunt and before starting their gardens or building their homes. They had other ceremonies of thanksgiving after the kill and at harvest time. They were aware of the Rhythm of Reciprocity and Generosity, and intentionally gave back with their gratitude, their time, and their ceremonies. Many indigenous cultures consciously rotated their hunting and fishing grounds and their use of natural resources to allow the earth time and space for restoration and renewal.

The Mayans believe that it pleases the gods to see beauty and to hear human beings laugh and sing. They intentionally made themselves beautiful, and created beauty in their lives with their clothing, tools, and ceremonies as a way to give back to the gods for the gift of life in a human body.

Gratitude is the experience of acknowledgment for a gift that has been given. It is part of the Rhythm of Reciprocity and Generosity.

How Can We Practice Reciprocity and Generosity?

There are many ways to bring reciprocity and gratitude into our daily living.

- We can tithe or set aside a set amount of our income to regularly give to charity or to projects that support or nourish us spiritually.

- We can keep a Gratitude Journal in which, each night before sleep, we write three things for which we are grateful.

- We can pause before eating a meal and think or speak aloud words of gratitude for all who contributed to bringing us this nourishment so necessary for sustaining our life. Another way to bring greater awareness of the gift of food is to consciously savor the first mouthful.

- Some people's reciprocity practice is to pick up trash where they walk. Others work in community projects. Still others work with animal or plant rescue missions.

- We can practice acknowledgment, and create ceremonies to express gratitude for gifts such as good health, new endeavors, achievements, friendship, and more.

I have a gratitude practice when I receive a patient's payment at the end of their appointment. We both hold onto the money as I say, "Bless the Creator and all who touch this. May it return to us ten thousand times and bring with it healing and peace. And believing this to be so, so be it." As soon as I say this, I experience the whole atmosphere around the money shifting from one of uncomfortable necessity to a sense of gracious ease and joy.

I once had a patient who forgot to bring his checkbook and so couldn't pay

PRACTICING RECIPROCITY

Donate to charities or projects that support you spiritually/tithe

✦

Keep a Gratitude Journal

✦

Speak your gratitude before meals, and savor the first mouthful

✦

Help your community as you can (even picking up trash helps out)

✦

Practice acknowledgment and appreciation

✦

Create ceremonies to express gratitude for gifts (good health, friends, etc.)

✦

Give thanks when exchanging money for services

me at the time of the visit. Later, I received his check in the mail with a note that read, "Don't worry, Dr. Rothschild, I've already blessed the check."

What Is the Relation between Generosity and the Experience of Health?

Generosity means approaching life with a "yes" rather than a "no." When we speak a "yes," the heart opens; and when we speak a "no," it closes. Generosity is open-heartedness, kindness of spirit, compassion.

Someone I knew once told me, "If you are gifting someone something of yours, always give the best one. That way you have given them the best one; and once it is gone, you will still have the best one of those that remain."

In practicing generosity, do not forget to include yourself. Be generous, kind, and compassionate to yourself in your thoughts as well as your actions.

DANCING WITH ALL THESE RHYTHMS

As we grow in our awareness of these universal Principles, Rhythms, and Cycles, we can begin to practice harmonizing with them. Of course, not all aspects of our life may be in the same rhythm or cycle. We can be in different rhythms at the same time. For example, our new creative venture may be in the seasonal energy of Spring and new beginnings, while simultaneously our day job may be in a full-tilt boogie in the height of Summer energy, and our love relationship may be gestating deep in Winter stillness. Meanwhile, our plans for travel may be in the Transition stage of creation, requiring our focus and attention in short, powerful bursts.

Some elements in our life may be flowering, while others are fruiting and some are dying. Use your knowledge of these rhythms and cycles to identify what is going on at times when you feel unclear and cannot see the way forward. If you can identify the rhythm, you can find your own unique way to dance with it.

Allow space and time to assess what is going on before moving into action or reaction. Ask yourself, "How is the Rhythm of Reciprocity and Generosity manifesting in my life?" "Am I holding myself and others with compassion and kindness?"

*Our lives and our health are intrinsically linked
with the web of life of this planet and all life on it.*

CHAPTER TWO

THE GOLDEN KEY

Engaging the Rhythm of Good Digestion

"Harmony with the rhythm of digestion is vital to achieving and maintaining health. Failure to acknowledge or support this rhythm undermines the body's natural inclination to balance and health. When we are in harmony with our digestive rhythm, we can optimize wellness and restore vitality." —MARIANNE ROTHSCHILD, M.D.

"In understanding the basics of digestion, you'll discover who's in charge. Here's a hint. It's not you." —NANCY S. MURE

Good digestion is a fundamental key to health. Just as a car cannot drive if its engine is unable to use its fuel, a body that cannot digest food properly will always be compromised. If the body lacks a healthy working ability to break down and assimilate food, good health is impossible to achieve and maintain. Even if we take additional vitamin and nutritional supplements, it is unlikely that much of these are actually absorbed if we cannot digest food well. We need to engage with the Rhythms of Good Digestion.

HOW DOES GOOD DIGESTION HAPPEN?

The whole process of digestion actually begins when we smell food cooking. Who hasn't enjoyed the aroma of onions cooking, bacon frying, or bread fresh from the oven? The smell of food stimulates the salivary glands in the mouth to start secreting enzyme-rich saliva. Ever notice that if you chew a mouthful of rice or crackers long enough, it begins to taste sweet?

That is because the saliva contains enzymes that digest carbohydrates and break them down into simple sugars.

When we begin to chew our food, the act of chewing initiates the release of hydrochloric acid in the stomach. This acid is necessary and vital to break down bulky proteins into smaller particles. It also allows minerals to be separated into ionic particles, which makes them available to be absorbed. Stomach acid also stimulates the release of other enzymes, such as *pepsin* and *gastrin*, to further digest proteins, as well as *Intrinsic Factor*, which must combine with Vitamin B12 before it can be absorbed. Once the acidified food bolus, or mass, moves to the small intestines, the gallbladder and pancreas are triggered to contribute their secretions to digestion. The gallbladder squeezes out a load of bile to help break down the fats, and the pancreas sends enzymes that further break down fats and carbohydrates.

At this point, we already can see a number of ways in which our current habits around food may be compromising our digestion process. If we are rarely around food while it's cooking and therefore don't get to *smell* it, our salivary glands don't get a warm-up. And if we don't eat food that requires a bit of *chewing*, stomach-acid production may be compromised. If we are just sipping smoothies or downing so-called energy bars or a few bites of yogurt, we may not adequately trigger our digestive process into action.

The digestive process is also compromised if we drink copious amounts of liquids (water, tea, soda, etc.) *with* our meal. Liquids dilute our stomach acid and make it less effective. *Ice-cold* liquids reduce the stomach's enzymatic activity even further. Ideally, the amount of additional liquids drunk should be kept to four ounces or less during a meal and up to an hour afterwards. Drinking less with a meal has other benefits as well. It may take us more time to eat. Food may need to be chewed longer in order to generate enough saliva so that it can be easy to swallow. Eating more slowly helps digestion and gives time for our satiety bell to ring and let us know we have eaten enough.

In summary, digestion is quite a complicated process and there are many ways that it can be disturbed:

▪ If we are not *present for the cooking smells*... then we miss activating our salivary glands. Our initial digestive activity is thwarted.

- If we don't *chew our food*, or don't *eat food that requires chewing…* then we don't fully activate our stomach acid and its retinue of enzymes and Intrinsic Factor.

- Without *adequate stomach acid…* the minerals in foods cannot be split into ionic particles for absorption.

- If we dilute our stomach acid with large amounts of liquids when we eat… then the stomach acid is less effective.

- If we are taking an acid-blocker like Zantac or Propulsid or similar products that reduce or eliminate stomach-acid production… then we cannot break down food into smaller particles, or turn the minerals into absorbable forms, or secrete Intrinsic Factor to bind with Vitamin B12.

- If the food bolus (mass) is not properly acidified when it enters the small intestine… then the gallbladder and pancreatic functions are compromised, which affects fat and carbohydrate digestion and absorption.

- If our gallbladder is not working well… then we may lack sufficient bile to break down fats adequately.

The end result of a digestive system that isn't working well is that we are not getting the nutrients we need for optimal health. Even if we take additional vitamin and nutritional supplements, it is unlikely that much of these are actually absorbed.

DIGESTION AND THE MIND-BODY CONNECTION

Many things influence how our digestion works. Our nervous system is a major influence. If we are constantly in "fight or flight" mode—all run and no rest, anxious, or stressed out—then we are in Sympathetic Nervous System overdrive. The Sympathetic Nervous System controls the body's responses to a perceived threat and is responsible for the "fight-or-flight" response. Here, the body speeds up, tenses up, and becomes more alert, and the functions not essential for survival are shut down.

Its counterpart, the Parasympathetic Nervous System, controls homeostasis and the body at rest, and is responsible for the body's "rest-and-digest" function, restoring the body to a state of calm and relaxation.

When the Sympathetic Nervous System is activated, the Parasympathetic Nervous System is automatically turned off.

This is unfortunate, because it is the *Parasympathetic* Nervous system that stimulates our restorative processes, which include digestion, reproduction, and sleep. It has been noted that the birthing process (governed by the Parasympathetic Nervous System) will cease in a laboring animal if she becomes frightened or feels threatened. Her contractions will simply stop. I know of women who experienced strong labor contractions while they were still at home, yet these completely stopped when they got to the hospital—perhaps because it was an unfamiliar surrounding and they felt scared.

Someone who is constantly in "fight or flight" mode is in Sympathetic Nervous System overdrive, and spends little time dancing in the more restorative rhythm of the Parasympathetic Nervous System. Our culture's hyper-busy stressful pace of life often means that most people's digestive systems have difficulty maintaining normal activity. Most people consider one bowel movement a day "a good day." But the ideal is *one bowel movement after every meal.*

To support our digestion, we need to engage the Parasympathetic Nervous System; and so when we eat, we need to consciously stop being fast-paced and still ourselves. It may help to take a few deep breaths before taking the first bite, and to offer thanks for the nourishment about to enter our body. Being more present when eating directly helps to turn on the Parasympathetic Nervous system, whereas eating while driving or working at our desk may not have the same effect.

YOUR NERVOUS SYSTEM(S) AT A GLANCE

Sympathetic Nervous System —"Fight or Flight" (alert, adrenaline activation, functions not essential for survival shut down)

Parasympathetic Nervous System —"Rest and Digest" (calm and relaxation; stimulates the body's restorative processes, such as digestion, reproduction, sleep)

A colleague of mine took a trip to Spain and noted her findings in her blog. She found it quite curious that Spaniards have greater longevity than many other Europeans, yet they eat fat, drink wine, and smoke. I think one piece of the puzzle is that the Spanish still observe their custom of *siesta* almost religiously. After a hearty midday meal, shops close and people retreat to rest—which supports good digestion. Shops and activity resume later in the day and continue into the evening. Could the siesta be the secret to their longevity and apparent good health? A pause after a big meal certainly supports *the Rhythm of Digestion*. It also supports *the Rhythm of Rejuvenation*—balancing work with rest.

ONE WOMAN'S JOURNEY BACK TO HEALTH

"You are my last hope," Nora said, carefully lowering herself into the chair beside my desk. "I know every bathroom in town, all too well."

Her words told me that she had already been on her journey to health for some time. I settled back in my chair. "Tell me your story," I requested with genuine interest. "Begin at the beginning."

Digestive trouble had plagued Nora for over 30 years. For many of those years, she had attempted to manage it with over-the-counter remedies, antacids, lactaid, beano, senna, Imodium, and more. All the while, she was maintaining an action-packed life as a wife and mother, as well as holding down a full-time job—a lifestyle that many women find themselves living these days. Now in her 50s with her children grown and on their own, Nora had time to focus on her digestion problems and she wanted to resolve them.

She had begun her journey with her primary-care physician, who had tried a few things such as prescription antacids and constipation aids, but they hadn't helped. Her doctor then referred her to a specialist—a gastroenterologist who had performed the almost obligatory endoscopy and colonoscopy, with the result that nothing out of the ordinary was discovered. He had noted some redness ("erythema" is the medical term) or swelling ("edema") in Nora's esophagus and stomach. In the end, the doctor had given her a diagnosis of GERD, or Gastroesophageal Reflux, and Irritable Bowel Syndrome. At his recommendation, she tried stronger prescription medications for suppressing stomach acid, but still there was no relief of her symptoms. Additional prescription drugs to improve her alternating constipation and diarrhea produced little improvement. Eventually, she tried antidepressants and anti-anxiety medications. Nothing seemed to help.

By the time Nora first came to see me, she was experiencing explosive diarrhea: four or more episodes in the morning, and randomly through her day. She noted significant bloating and a sensation of fullness in her abdomen after eating. This grew worse as the day progressed, even though she limited herself to eating small amounts at a time. Often when she lay down at night, she experienced burning and discomfort in her lower chest. All this despite the fact that she was currently taking one of the more powerful prescription proton-pump inhibitors, a drug designed to turn off stomach-acid production. She was also having trouble sleeping well, and noted that her energy had begun to flag in the past few years.

Her life revolved around her poor digestion. She had to wait until she felt safe to leave home (and her own bathroom) in the morning. She knew every public bathroom in town. She rarely was able to enjoy a meal with friends for fear of discomfort or disastrous embarrassing consequences.

"I really hope you can help me," Nora concluded, a tense smile on her face. "I'm so desperate for relief and a life worth living."

"It sounds like these problems have made living a full life very difficult for you," I responded. "The good news is that I have been able to help many people who suffered from similar difficulties."

Nora's face momentarily brightened.

"Tell me about your health as a child and growing up."

"Even as a kid I had sort of a nervous stomach...." Nora continued her story.

After she had completed her story, I examined her. Her blood pressure was low, as was her temperature. She was rather thin, with a sallow tint to her skin and lack of luster in her hair. There were circles under her eyes and her tongue was pale with a greasy, whitish coat. She had no swelling or edema in her hands or feet, When I palpated her belly, I found no sign of enlarged liver or spleen and only a slight tenderness below the ribcage in the middle, where her stomach was. When I pressed firmly in the area up under her right ribcage, she did not experience pain. Had there been discomfort or pain in this area, I might suspect that her gallbladder was irritated or inflamed. In addition, Nora did not recall that her symptoms only started an hour or so after a meal. (More about gallbladder issues later in this chapter.)

Looking for the Causative Conditions

Fundamental to my holistic understanding of illness is that the symptoms that show up in the present are often the accumulated effect of many different issues that have piled up over time. Nora's initial digestion problem had expressed itself as diarrhea. Years of diarrhea and antacid use had diminished her body's ability to absorb nutrients. The resulting nutrient deficiencies had, in turn, produced still other symptoms and problems.

As I examined Nora, I mentally reviewed the many possible explanations for her problems. *Let's see,* I thought. *She may have food sensitivities.* I considered the dark circles under her eyes: *That may indicate chronic sinus congestion, a common symptom resulting from allergies. She may have developed food allergies after the diarrhea washed away the bacteria that would have broken down food proteins before they entered the bloodstream.* And then there was her coated tongue: *Maybe indicative of a yeast overgrowth.* She might have acquired the bacteria *Clostridium difficile*—*although*, I reasoned, *it's possible her previous physicians already checked for that.* I shook my head and took a deep breath. To achieve lasting resolution, we would need to work through the layers of issues.

"It will take time to completely resolve your problem," I began. "There are a number of layers that we will need to work through—it's rather like peeling an onion."

Nora nodded thoughtfully, "Yes, I'm beginning to understand. So how do we begin?"

Exploring Treatments

In partnering with my patients on their journey to wellness, I need to be responsive to their capacity to adopt new ideas, because people approach change and challenges in many different ways. Some patients arrive in my office ready to dive right into a new lifestyle, and want to begin implementing all my suggestions immediately. Others want my opinion and suggestions, but are not quite ready to initiate any major changes. Some wait and return months or years later, when they are finally ready to make changes. Many people have other major time- and life-commitments that limit their ability to carry out a new treatment path. As their holistic health guide, part of my work is to discern what path and pace will have the greatest potential for success for each patient.

As I turned over in my mind the possible avenues of treatment, I also assessed how open Nora was to making some changes. I wanted to find some key interventions that would give her enough immediate relief to encourage her to keep working with me on the remaining symptoms. I used my understanding of the digestive process to make my choice of intervention.

In Nora's case, the diarrhea indicated that her body was moving food too quickly through her digestive tract—too quickly for nutrients to be absorbed well, and even to reabsorb enough fluid to produce a solid stool. In addition, the flushing action of diarrhea washes away the *good* bacteria that live on the tiny hairs (villi) that line the interior of our intestines. These resident gut bacteria function as the final and critical phase of digestion: they further break down large macromolecules, such as proteins, into smaller molecules, which then can pass through the semi-permeable membrane of the capillary walls that line the gut into the bloodstream and into the body to supply the nutrients needed for health.

"Do your symptoms improve when you use antacids?" I asked her. I was starting to wonder if Nora could have a deficiency in stomach-acid production.

"No," she answered, "not even when I use the strongest ones—those proton-pump inhibitors."

So I suggested, "Maybe part of your digestive problem is that you are not making enough stomach acid, and that's why blocking acid production didn't improve things." I elaborated, "Most people, including doctors, believe that GERD is only caused by *too much* stomach acid. But at least half the people I have seen with heartburn or reflux symptoms are not over-producing stomach acid. They actually *don't make enough stomach acid* to facilitate food breakdown."

Nora's widened eyes showed that she was all ears.

"Between the esophagus and the stomach," I continued, "is the lower esophageal sphincter. If food washes up out of the stomach into the esophagus, we get typical GERD symptoms like a burning sensation. But the lower esophageal sphincter is not a typical sphincter muscle, like your anus. It is an area that is extremely sensitive to pH or acidity. If the stomach is not sufficiently *acidified*, the sphincter doesn't close, and acid can wash into the esophagus."

We tend to make less stomach acid as we age. However, the inadequate production of stomach acid can afflict younger people, as well, even teenagers. Some people don't have enough of the prerequisite nutrients, such as zinc, needed to *make* stomach acid. Zinc and magnesium deficiencies are very common these days.

This line of reasoning led me to a potential treatment for Nora. "When people who don't make enough stomach acid take additional Betaine HCl with each meal," I told her, "their symptoms resolve."

"What's Betaine HCl?" Nora asked.

"It's Betaine Hydrochloride, the same acid as the hydrochloric acid that our stomach makes," I explained. "It comes in capsules. You can find it where vitamins are sold."

She brightened visibly.

"Would you be willing to take a simple test to determine whether your stomach-acid production is adequate?" I asked her.

"*Would* I?" she responded. "Absolutely!" She seemed eager to try something—anything!

"Okay, then!" I smiled.

The Stomach Acid Test

I reviewed with her how to do a simple trial by taking one capsule of Betaine HCl during or immediately after a meal. If she experienced a burning sensation in her stomach within 30 minutes or less, this would mean that her body made enough stomach acid when she ate, and now there was too much. The burning would resolve immediately after she drank four ounces of water mixed with two teaspoons of baking soda. However, if she *did not* feel any burning in 30 minutes, then we could conclude that she *did not* make enough stomach acid.

"If you do not experience burning, you need to continue to take the Betaine HCl with every meal," I concluded.

"Will I need to take it for the rest of my life?" Nora was sounding a bit concerned, now. Not many people relish the idea of needing to take a pill forever.

"For some people, that means for the rest of their lives. But many others find that after taking Betaine HCl for some months or years, they start to experience a burning sensation after they take it. This suggests that the Betaine HCl helped them to rebuild their mineral stores and now they can make adequate stomach acid on their own. At that point, they no longer need to supplement their stomach acid."

Drinking Water

Nora had told me that she drank four to six quarts of water a day, so I added, "Many people unknowingly dilute their stomach acid by drinking large quantities of liquids with their meals. Ice-cold drinks are especially hard on the digestive process." I suggested that she limit the amount of liquid drunk at a meal to four ounces or less, and drink her liquids an hour or more *after* meals, once her stomach had emptied. She agreed to this.

Since Nora's problem might be that she was not making enough stomach acid, I decided to start with a few key changes and see what happened. The first change was to try Betaine HCl and see if it helped. If she experienced no burning sensation, then she was to continue to take it with each meal. If she did experience burning within a half hour after taking the Betaine HCl, she would switch to taking digestive enzymes that did not contain the acid.

Eliminating Wheat

I didn't want to overwhelm Nora with too many lifestyle changes all at once, so I asked if she thought she could handle a second intervention.

"Sure," she said. "What do I have to lose?"

So I told her, "I noticed from your food diary that many of the foods you eat have wheat in them." Together we looked at her food diary. I took a yellow highlighter and marked the foods she ate that contained wheat—such as granola bars, crackers, breads, and cereals.

"What's wrong with wheat?" she asked me.

"Today's wheat is different from the wheat that your grandma and grandpa ate," I explained. "I grew up in Kansas, and I remember the beautiful wheat fields, with their long, tall, pale-gold stalks and large seedheads. Sometimes, just before harvest time, a big storm would come, and those big heads would fill with water and the whole field of sodden wheat would be flattened—the stalks were unable to bear the weight. A farmer could lose his whole harvest in a single night.

"But not anymore. In the 1960s and '70s," I continued, "scientists began using hybridization methods to develop a new kind of wheat. The farmers wanted smaller heads and the bakers wanted more gluten. Today's wheat is much shorter, with smaller heads on top. When I see wheat growing in the field today, it is a dark-brownish color and about 18 to 22 inches tall. Gone are the waving fields of pale gold that I remember from childhood. This new wheat won't be destroyed by a late-season storm, which translates into less risk for the farmers. It has also been designed specifically to have more gluten, which makes the bakers happy. But it is much harder on the digestive systems of the people who eat it."

I checked to see if Nora was still listening. She was sitting very quietly, watching me intently.

"In addition," I explained, "this newly engineered wheat contains hundreds of unique compounds that we humans have never encountered before—and our bodies are responding differently to it. And it's not only humans who are having problems: according to reports, even *pigs* are having digestive problems with the new wheat. Today's wheat is highly inflammatory.

"This is the wheat that is grown today, worldwide. Only small pockets of the older strains are still grown, nowadays—in southern France, parts of Italy, and the Middle East. If you want more details about how wheat has changed and how that is affecting human beings, Dr. William Davis has written extensively on this in his books, *Wheatbelly* and *The Wheatbelly Cookbook*."

Nora's eyes had widened considerably, a sign that she was really taking in what I was saying. I decided to share some of my own story about wheat with her, so that she had something real and personal to relate to (and to let her know that I was once on the same journey as she was on now).

"My own journey with wheat began," I told her, "when I noticed that I would experience a mental fog and physical sluggishness after eating pasta. Over time, I chose to eat less and less pasta. When I stopped eating pasta entirely, I found that I could feel full and satisfied without the heavy feeling in my belly that pasta seemed to create. And then I noticed the same heavy feeling after eating pizza, so I ate less pizza. Then I began to leave out bread, and found other ways of eating without resorting to toast or sandwiches. About a year or two ago, I stopped eating *all* grains, as well as beans and starchy vegetables. I wanted to see how I felt."

"And…?" Nora prompted me.

"That's when I noticed the biggest change," I said brightly. "Not only was my mind clearer, but I also had a more sustained energy, and my whole body felt somehow lighter, more lithe. I noticed that my clothes became looser. Today, I eat some corn, and if I want bread I use the flat German sourdough rye bread."

"That's a very persuasive recommendation," Nora said enthusiastically. "I'm ready to make changes!"

"That's great!" I smiled. "So my second recommendation is that you a*void all wheat* for at least a month. It can take up to a month to see the full effect of a wheat-free diet." I instructed her, "You'll need to read the *Ingredients* list on any packaged foods in order to discover if there is wheat in what you're eating. Don't confuse the Ingredients list with the *Nutritional Facts* list, which is also on the label. And you will need to avoid the bread, breading, and gravies in restaurant food and in prepared foods, as they commonly contain wheat."

I wanted Nora to leave stocked with sufficient interventions to make a difference in her wellbeing, but not feeling that the changes were too challenging. So I checked in with her. "How does that sound to you? Does it sound overwhelming?"

"No," Nora laughed, "it sounds…exciting! I once tried to eliminate wheat in the past, but only for a week at most. And I wasn't sure if it helped."

Eating Cooked Foods

Since she seemed so enthusiastic to try new ways, I decided to risk a third suggestion: "My final recommendation is to *eat only cooked food*. Cooking helps break down food and make it more digestible," I explained. "It gives your body a break, and promotes gut healing."

A cooked-foods diet is especially important when there is clear evidence that digestion is not going well (such as diarrhea, abdominal pain, bloating). I suggested to Nora that she eat nothing raw or even cold. "Fruits as well as vegetables must be cooked. They can be poached, sautéed, or baked. Salad greens can be placed at the bottom of a bowl of hot soup, where they will quickly turn soft and cook."

I knew first-hand about the wisdom of eating only cooked foods. When I was ten, my parents took my younger brother and me to Europe for the summer. One day, my father fainted right in the middle of the Piazza de San Marco in Venice. It seems he had come down with a stomach bug. For the next five days, we stayed close to our hotel as my father lay in bed and recovered. The hotel brought up big tureens of risotto, a concoction of arborio rice cooked for hours in chicken broth. They knew that a weak digestion needed well-cooked foods. I can personally attest to the delicious flavor of the risotto (my father could only eat a little and so I obligingly helped out).

The Chinese have taken this idea of slow-cooked food—they call it *congee*—and made it into a highly sophisticated healing art. There are many books that contain hundreds of different congee recipes—various combinations of rice or other grains, herbs, vegetables, meats, and broths, each designed to treat a specific medical condition. I have heard that in traditional Chinese hospitals, patients are accompanied by family members who stay and cook for them according to the doctors' explicit instructions. (Hospital patients also supply their own bedding, including pajamas—which sounds like a vast improvement over what patients experience in most hospitals here in the U.S.!)

I once had a gentleman in his seventies who came to me for a terrible problem with diarrhea. If he ate anything at all, his diarrhea would begin and not stop. The problem had become increasingly unmanageable over the past three years. His biggest upset was that he could no longer take his granddaughter out to eat—an activity they had often enjoyed together. His wife had died some years ago, and he had no idea how to cook anything. He survived on packaged foods and restaurant fare.

I began by teaching him some basic cooking skills. At my suggestion, he acquired a crockpot. I instructed him to fill it with water and a tablespoon of vinegar; add a chicken (including bones, and preferably with the skin still on it); cut up celery, onion, and carrots; add some rice, salt, and pepper; and let it cook at a low temperature for four to six hours at least. This was ALL he was to eat for breakfast, lunch, dinner, and snacks. He could make several different versions, using beef, fish, lamb, or pork. But nothing raw; no breads, crackers, or chips; and no milk products. He could eat fruit, provided it was cooked.

After having survived three years of terrible diarrhea, the poor man was so desperate that he followed my instructions to a T. It took some time for him to heal. However, by the end of a year, his diarrhea had disappeared and his energy had returned. He and his granddaughter resumed their outings. And, as a bonus benefit, he had learned how to cook for himself.

I have had many clients experience favorable changes after integrating my suggestions for improving their digestion. I hoped Nora would soon be one of them. I had checked with her to make sure that she was ready, willing, and able to make some major lifestyle changes, and she had assured me she was.

Nora left with her three instructions: (1) try Betaine HCl and continue taking it each meal, if it didn't burn, (2) avoid wheat, and (3) only eat food that is cooked.

"Come back in a week," I told her. "I hope you get to bring good news."

A week later, she returned to report on her results. "I can't believe it!" she said. "The diarrhea is *gone* and I've had no heartburn. I haven't felt this good in years!" She was thrilled with her progress—and so was I. She had managed to make her own congees or stews with various meats and vegetables, and found them quite palatable. Most of all, she was encouraged that she was on the right track at last.

"Let's meet again in six weeks," I suggested. "That will give us some time to see the effect of removing wheat from your diet. Meanwhile, continue to eat only cooked foods, and stay off the acid-blocker medication."

So what was the result of Nora's willing experiment? Six weeks later she returned to report, "Not only is my diarrhea gone for the first time in years, but I seem to have more energy! And my mind seems clearer."

"That's wonderful!" I said, beaming. I felt as excited as she was.

GALLBLADDER PROBLEMS

It seemed that Nora was justifiably confident in her new way of eating, but she had another question. "Should I worry about my gallbladder?" Her brow wrinkled as she explained, "Most of the women in my family—including my grandmother, my mother, and her sister—have had their gallbladders removed."

"That's not an uncommon story," I responded. "Surgical removal of the gallbladder is often medically advised. But it can come at a price. When I examined you at our first appointment, you had no pain when I pressed deeply under your right rib cage, where your gallbladder is. Tenderness in that area can indicate that your gallbladder is inflamed."

"But I want to avoid the same fate as the other women in my family," she persisted. "I would like to keep my gallbladder, if possible."

"Yes, of course," I agreed. "The key is to make sure that there is enough fat and vegetables in your diet to keep the gallbladder active. A diet that is super-low in fat and fiber fails to properly stimulate the gallbladder, and the bile stored in it becomes stagnant and may turn into stones or sludge. So make sure you cook those vegetables with plenty of fat." (The kinds of fats that are good to cook with are discussed in detail in Chapter Three: Nutrition—Finding Your *Nourishing* Rhythm.)

The gallbladder is a small, hollow organ tucked under the liver. It stores bile, which is made in the liver. Bile is a yellow-brown-greenish bitter fluid that breaks down fats. After food has been partially digested in the stomach, it then moves through the pyloric valve into the small intestines. This movement stimulates the gallbladder to contract, and a bolus of bile passes through the bile duct into the small intestines, where it breaks down the fats in the food bolus.

In medical school, I was taught that women who were "fat, fertile, and forty" were prime candidates for gallbladder problems. Gallbladder problems seem to affect women much more than men, and often begin around the age of forty. Someone whose gallbladder is not working very well can experience pain when it constricts to send bile to the intestines.

Rosa was a patient with long-standing gallbladder issues. When I examined her, she winced when I pressed deeply under her right ribcage. "That's exactly where I feel the pain," she told me. "When I went to my primary-care doctor about the pain, he told me to just avoid eating fats or to get my gallbladder removed. But I know fats are good for you, so I want to be able to eat them."

I agreed with her. "The problem with avoiding fats in the diet is it's not healthy. And by decreasing the work for the gallbladder, we have not resolved its dysfunction, but merely are hoping to avoid it." Rosa nodded in agreement.

Going further into Rosa's concern, I inquired, "Have you had an ultrasound study done on your gallbladder?"

Often, doctors will order tests such as an ultrasound to determine if the gallbladder contains gallstones or "sludge." Another test that can be ordered is a HIDA scan. Here, a radioactive tracer is injected into the blood, and—through a nuclear medicine scanner—the movement of the bile through the liver, gallbladder, and bile ducts is observed. The HIDA scan may show that the poor gallbladder barely contracts, or appears completely shriveled up.

"Yes," she replied. "My ultrasound showed sludge in the gallbladder. But I'd really like to avoid surgery. Almost every woman in my family has had their gallbladder removed, and now they have to be really careful about what they eat."

I have heard this from a number of women. Their mothers, grandmothers, aunts, and sisters all had gallbladder problems and all ended up having surgery. Is that so bad? No, but it is not my first choice for a solution to the problem of a weak gallbladder. Whether there is some genetic predisposition or whether families simply tend to make similar food choices is something for geneticists and epidemiologists to determine. I know a number of women who have broken with family tradition and maintained a healthy gallbladder through a good diet and using bile salts, if needed.

In addition to reducing the body's ability to digest fats, surgery does not always resolve the pain problem. I have seen some people whose pain continued to be a problem, even after surgery removed their gallbladder.

"What can I do to avoid gallbladder surgery?" Rosa looked at me imploringly.

"If your gallbladder is weak and you get pain when you eat fats," I began, "then you need to take bile salts with your meal to supplement what the gallbladder cannot produce. I have recommended bile salts as a mealtime supplement for many women (and men) with gallbladder pain and problems. The bile salts helped them manage to keep their gallbladders as well as stop having pain."

If your gallbladder is weak and you get pain when
you eat fats, then for the time being you need to
take bile salts with your meal to supplement what
the gallbladder cannot produce.

One patient of mine with a touchy gallbladder always knew when it was time to start taking the bile-salts supplements again, because she would feel pain in her gallbladder while horseback riding. Pregnancy also can aggravate a weak gallbladder, perhaps because the hormones of pregnancy seem to relax smooth muscle, which may make the gallbladder function less efficiently. With the help of bile salts, my equestrian patient made it through seven pregnancies and managed to keep her gallbladder until the eighth.

Prevention is always the best choice. If you eat meals that routinely contain a reasonable amount of fat as well as fiber (that means vegetables), the gallbladder will be exercising its squeezing action regularly. Bile won't tend to collect to become sludge or gallstones. Remember, fats are not the enemy; they are an essential nutrient and an important part of a healthy diet.

Gallstones *can* dissolve: supplements such as Vitamin B6 and folate can help, in many cases. It has also been found helpful to identify any food allergies, and eliminate those foods from your diet. Surgery should be considered as a *last* resort, after all other approaches have failed.

I told Rosa, "Avoiding fats doesn't really help the gallbladder return to healthy functioning. Today's low-fat craze may actually be contributing to the problem. And fats are a very important food group. Butter, for example, contains very important fat-soluble vitamins, such as A, D, and K."

Leaky Gut Syndrome

When Nora returned for her three-month appointment, she announced triumphantly, "I'm doing much better!" Then grinning, she added, "The only time the diarrhea returned was when I cheated and had some birthday cake and ice cream. Boy, did I pay for that! It took almost a week before I was back to normal."

She pulled out her notebook. "I've been doing some reading, and I have some questions. Do I have 'Leaky Gut Syndrome'?"

"Leaky Gut Syndrome" has recently been getting a lot of publicity as the new title for gut dysbiosis. It can develop after taking one or several rounds of antibiotics, or after one or more bouts of diarrhea. The result is that the normal population, or "biome," of bacteria and yeasts that live on the hair-like villi of the small intestine are killed or washed away. In their wake, other less helpful bacteria and yeasts have taken their place. (Kind of like crabgrass taking over your lawn.) These invaders do not perform the final digestive breakdown, as the desirable flora do. The end result is that larger food particles—including large food-protein molecules—pass intact from the gut into the bloodstream. The digestive capacity of the gut has been compromised, and the gut has become "leaky."

Inside the bloodstream is our internal "Homeland Security System"—part of the body's immune system. Its function is to seek out foreign proteins, such as invading viruses or bacteria, and destroy them. Once "Homeland Security" has identified a specific foreign invader (such as the measles or chicken-pox virus, for example), it creates specific antibodies to them, which remain on patrol in the bloodstream for months or years. As a result, it is able to mount a powerful response when a repeat exposure occurs. The immune system uses a number of different defense mechanisms, many of which involve creating inflammation.

When the gut lacks the appropriate bacteria to fully break down the food proteins, they pass directly into the bloodstream as large macromolecules. These large food proteins may include casein (from milk), albumin (from egg whites), and gluten (from wheat, rye and a few other grains). Our "Homeland Security" identifies these large food macromolecules as "foreign proteins." As part of its normal defense response, it makes antibodies that are specific to the food proteins it finds in the blood. Antibodies such as IgG and IgA ("Ig" is the short way of writing Immunoglobulin) are produced that are specific for gluten, gliadin, albumin, casein, and other food proteins. These antibodies circulate in the blood (IgA can also be detected in the saliva). When a later exposure to these food proteins occurs in the blood, the antibodies initiate a whole cascade of immune responses, creating inflammation both in the gut and in other parts of the body.

Someone with 'Leaky Gut" (i.e., without sufficient gut bacteria to fully break down food proteins) will have specific antibodies for those foods circulating in their bloodstream. There are tests that one can use to determine if a person has IgG and IgA antibodies for specific foods and other entities. The inflammatory response that IgG and IgA trigger is a *delayed* reaction. It's important to know that the typical "food allergy panel" that conventional allergists use tests only for IgE, not for IgG or IgA. IgE is an antibody that mediates *immediate* reactions, such as hives or anaphylaxis. Most people are already aware of which foods give them an immediate allergic reaction.

Depending on which foods are commonly consumed, a person who has developed a leaky gut may have large amounts of food-protein mac-romolecules bobbing around in their bloodstream. These proteins may include gluten and gliadin (from wheat and other high-gluten grains), albumin (egg protein), casein (milk protein), or genistein (soy protein).

When I initially examined Nora, she had a coated tongue, indicat-ing that she had digestion problems. Three months later, her tongue still appeared coated. A coated tongue could signify an overgrowth of yeast. (There is a detailed discussion about candida, or yeast overgrowth, later in this chapter.)

After we examined her tongue, Nora said, "Well, I guess this proves that I still have digestion problems. How can we test for Leaky Gut syn-drome?"

I appreciated her courageous, collaborative spirit. "There are a number of good tests to determine whether you have yeast or abnormal bacteria or parasites," I began. (Laboratories that perform these tests are listed in the Appendix.) "There are also good tests for food allergies or sensitivities."

"We want to test for IgG and IgA, the antibodies that produce delayed reactions. Delayed reactions can take hours to days to appear. They can produce digestive symptoms such as bloating, inflammation, abdom-inal pain, and diarrhea, as well as other symptoms in other parts of the body, such as eczema and asthma."

HOW FOOD SENSITIVITIES OR FOOD ALLERGIES DEVELOP

Inside our bloodstream, as mentioned, our immune system is on patrol. Like Homeland Security, its job is to search out, identify, and destroy foreign invaders—macromolecular proteins that might be invading viruses or bacteria. Once the immune system has been exposed to a particular foreign protein (the polio virus, for example), it produces specific antibodies to that protein. If, at a later time, the body is exposed to the polio virus again, those pre-existing polio antibodies in the bloodstream immediately go into action. They trigger an alarm, and the whole immune system reacts. The result is a huge inflammatory response—mast cells break down and release histamine, which causes swelling and heat, and white cells rush to the scene to kill and remove the invaders. The purpose of the inflammatory response is to surround and destroy the invading protein before it can multiply and spread within the body.

In the case of Leaky Gut Syndrome, large food-protein molecules are passing intact into the bloodstream. Our Homeland Security immune system identifies them as foreign-invader proteins, and makes antibodies to them. At the next encounter with those food proteins, the immune system is now primed to create lots of inflammation. Once our immune system has developed antibodies to specific foods, we will experience symptoms of inflammation when we eat those foods. If we eat them frequently, our body remains in a constant state of inflammation.

Since the Standard American Diet (SAD) is largely composed of wheat, milk products, and eggs, many Americans who develop Leaky Gut Syndrome are likely to have antibodies to those specific food (wheat, milk, and egg) proteins in their blood. If they continue to eat a SAD diet, their bodies are in a constant state of inflammation. (More information on the SAD diet is found in Chapter Three: Nutrition—Finding Your *Nourishing* Rhythm.)

Nora looked pensive, taking this all in. "Was my diarrhea because of Leaky Gut Syndrome?" she asked me.

"Well," I responded, "it's not so easy to determine the *single* factor. When you eliminated wheat, your symptoms quieted down. And when you ate the birthday cake, which had wheat in it, they flared up again. You may have developed antibodies to gluten due to a leaky gut. However, eating only cooked foods also calmed down your digestion. And you added hydrochloric acid. So I don't have a simple answer for why your diarrhea stopped. It may have been the combination of all three interventions."

After taking in this information, Nora had another question. "I've been reading a lot about inflammation. What determines where inflammation occurs?"

"I don't know if anyone has the full answer to that," I admitted. "It may be that the weakest, most vulnerable system is affected. Or perhaps when the level of inflammation is very high, symptoms develop *all over the body.*"

The holistic perspective on inflammation is totally missed in conventional Western medicine, which has divided the body into sections, each one treated by a different specialist. When inflammation is in the *lungs*, pulmonologists call it "asthma" or "chronic bronchitis." When it's in the *skin*, dermatologists term it "eczema" or "dermatitis." In the *bladder*, it's diagnosed by urologists as "interstitial cystitis." In the *head*, the otolaryngologists diagnose "chronic sinusitis," "chronic rhinitis," or "chronic serous otitis." In the *gut*, gastroenterologists name it "reflux," "irritable bowel syndrome," "colitis," "gastritis," or "esophagitis." In the *muscles*, the rheumatologists pronounce "fibromyalgia." Inflammation can also cause blurred vision, arthritis, nerve pain and paresthesia, headache, and impaired mentation. The point is that specialists are not trained to see the whole picture. They focus on prescribing medications for the specific condition they have identified.

It reminds me of the old story of the four blind men who happen upon an elephant. Each carefully examines one part of the animal and attempts to understand the nature of it. The one feeling the ear says, "It is thin and flat like an enormous leathery leaf." The one touching the trunk says, "No, it is like a giant snake, round and able to coil or straighten." The one touching the side says, "No, you are both wrong, it is like a wall—massive and impenetrable." And the one touching the leg says, "No, no, no, you are *all* wrong. It is like the trunk of a tree, solid and upright." Each of them is right; yet each has only a limited perspective and does not see the whole elephant.

When we step back and look at what is happening in the whole body, we see the common root of inflammation. Inflammation can have various origins, including Leaky Gut Syndrome. Further investigation is needed. Real resolution comes when we address the *root cause* rather than just attempt to mask the symptoms.

If Nora had returned at six weeks and reported that she still had a lot of abdominal discomfort, I might have suggested that she do a stool test to get a clearer picture of what bacteria, yeasts, and parasites lived in her gut. Or I might have suggested a food-allergy test, looking for IgG and IgA antibodies to foods she was still eating.

Testing: A Collaborative Decision

The decision of when and if to do tests is another that I make together with my patient. Some people want to do all the testing right at the beginning. Others would rather make lifestyle changes first and wait and see if the additional expense of testing is still warranted.

If we had tested and found that Nora had IgG or IgA antibodies to certain foods, I would have suggested that she eliminate those foods from her diet for about six months. It takes about six months for most of the antibodies to die off. If that turned out to be the cause of her diarrhea, then the diarrhea should stop after a month of strict avoidance. In addition, I would have recommended that she add probiotics and fermented foods to replant good bacteria and help heal her leaky gut. After six months, we would have reintroduced the eliminated foods *one at a time*, spaced at least three days apart, to identify which foods caused her digestive problems to reoccur. Because inflammatory symptoms may take a few days to develop, it is important to give at least three days between the reintroduction of each food. (More details on this and the full Food Allergy Elimination Diet protocol are available in the Appendix at the end of this book.)

Elimination Diets

If Nora had decided against submitting to blood tests for food allergies, I might have suggested an *elimination diet* as an alternative to blood tests. The most common elimination diet removes the seven most likely foods that cause inflammation: (1) dairy (milk products and eggs); (2) citrus; (3) wheat and corn; (4) sugar; (5) chocolate; (6) caffeine; and (7) artificial food colorants and additives. It is helpful to avoid soy as well, and all grains high in gluten. That includes rye, barley, spelt, kamut, and triticale. After a month on the elimination diet, most people experience significant, if not complete, relief—often they find not only that their digestive disorder resolves, but that other bothersome issues resolve, as well.

When I lead groups in seasonal cleanses, we eliminate these seven food groups for ten days. People report relief from snoring, stuffy nose, post-nasal drip, brain fog, sinusitis, muscle pain, bladder problems, and other issues. Why? Because all these symptoms are the result of inflammation. When the foods causing the inflammation are eliminated, the symptoms improve or resolve.

CANDIDA

Remember Nora's coated tongue? A coated tongue can indicate a variety of conditions. It can indicate illness, or it can be a sign of poor digestion. It can also indicate a systemic overgrowth of yeast—most commonly, *Candida albicans*. This condition, called "candida" or "candidiasis," is most commonly the result of antibiotic use. Sometimes a single round of antibiotics can kill enough of our residential bacteria and result in a yeast overgrowth.

In medical school, I was taught that systemic candidiasis only occurred in people with AIDS, because their immune system was out of order. Many doctors, including gastroenterologists, still believe that. In my experience, I have seen many people who do not have HIV or AIDS suffer from a yeast overgrowth.

Once an antibiotic kills a significant amount of our native bacteria, the yeast have no obstacles to restrain their growth. If you have ever used yeast in baking, you know that to activate it you put it in a bowl of warm water and add sugar. In a matter of minutes, the yeast begins to bubble and expand. Our bodies are huge reservoirs of warmth, water, and sugar (especially on the SAD diet). If our diet contains a lot of high-glycemic foods that create high blood-sugar, we have given the yeast everything it needs to grow abundantly.

High-glycemic foods are those that break down into glucose, or blood sugar, very quickly. These foods include not only sugar (in its various guises) but also foods containing flour, such as pasta and baked goods. High-glycemic foods raise blood sugar higher and faster than other foods. (The following chapter on Nutrition has more about high-glycemic foods and their effect on the body.)

Correcting candidiasis and returning the body's biome to balance involves three steps. First, we need to stop eating foods with a high glycemic index. Second, we need to reduce the yeast population, either with herbs or prescription drugs or both. Third, we need to replace the good gut-bacteria that was lost.

In Summary

The Rhythm of Digestion is vital, and a core pillar for achieving and maintaining health. Failure to support this rhythm undermines the body's natural inclination to balance and health. When we live in harmony with our digestive rhythms, we optimize wellness and restore vitality.

CHAPTER THREE

NUTRITION

Finding Your Nourishing Rhythm

"Let food be your medicine and medicine be your food." —HIPPOCRATES

"Find your personal food melody that you can dance to for the rest of your life." —MARIANNE ROTHSCHILD, M.D.

O nce we have established our Rhythm of Digestion, the nutrients in our food can be properly absorbed.

Our next step is to find our Nourishing Rhythm. We must choose food that will provide us the nourishment we need to support our health and vitality.

We *know* that food is important to our wellbeing. We *want* to be healthy and feel good. And yet there is so much confusion about food: What's good for you? What's bad for you? What's in, what's out? What's "natural"?

This chapter is designed to give you some solid and clear information that will help you make good choices about the food you eat.

NUTRITION VS. NOURISHMENT

Science is constantly discovering new information on nutrition, and as a result we are steadily bombarded by bits and pieces of ever-changing health facts (or factoids) in the news.

Remember when *fiber* was the big thing? It began when scientists announced that the amount of fiber people ate was important for their health. Then the food industry took that idea and went to town. Candy bars were pumped full of bran (husks) from oat or wheat or psyllium, and suddenly they became healthful *fiber bars*. Now people could feel better about rushing off in the morning munching on a candy bar because at least they were getting their fiber.

What *is* fiber? Ever seen fiber in the supermarket? (I haven't.) Fiber isn't a food in its own right; instead, it is found in the indigestible part of vegetables—the part that makes them chewy, such as the strings in the celery, asparagus, or parsley. When we eat fiber-rich foods, the fiber adds bulk to the stool, which makes for larger, easier bowel movements. We *do* need fiber—but not as ground-up husks jammed into a candy bar or pop tart. The fiber that's really helpful is found in eating fresh or cooked vegetables. Things we have to chew a bit. Grandma was right when she reminded us to "Eat your vegetables!"

Remember when *protein* was the big news? The food industry jumped on that and added soybean protein isolates, or whey, or whatever cheap source of protein they could find—and suddenly, candy bars became *protein bars*. Today there's a myriad of protein powders containing protein from egg, soy, whey, brown rice, pea, or who knows what next. All these proteins have been highly processed into powders that can break down easily into drinkable smoothies with enough added flavors and sweeteners to make them palatable. The food industry is really good at giving us quick-and-easy ways to feel like we are "doing the right thing."

Then science declared that *antioxidants* were helpful in fighting cancer. People learned that many fruits are rich in antioxidants. Lately, it seems like it's the "Fruit of the Month" club. Remember noni? Suddenly noni juice was key to good health. What *is* a noni? Ever see one growing? Then it was goji berries—"full of antioxidants, healthy." Where do these gogis grow anyway? Acerola, acai, pomegranates, noni, mangosteen—as each exotic new food is "discovered," the market fills with juices, dried powders, capsules, and more, all containing these wonder foods. Most of them have been highly processed, with sweeteners and flavorings added to make them more palatable. The processing has also destroyed much of the original valued ingredients.

It seems like every week, we hear news blasts about the amazing health benefits of some new discovery or another. No wonder our heads are spinning and we feel like we can't keep up with the information! There is so much information about nutrition. Yet I fear we have strayed ever deeper into a disconnect from our bodies and our nature.

The real question is: *What truly nourishes us?* Is our goal Nutrition or *Nourishment?* Wouldn't our own *bodies* know what nourishes us? If the food we are eating gives us energy, mental clarity, a body that moves without pain, good digestion, good rest, few illnesses, and a positive outlook—wouldn't you say that would be feedback that we are well nourished?

A HOLISTIC APPROACH TO EATING

"What diet should I be on?" was the first question out of Soraya's mouth as she plopped herself down in the chair at her initial appointment. "I want to lose weight and have more energy," she added, anxiously glancing up at me. A woman in her late forties, she was clearly overweight.

I can't tell you how many patients arrive asking this same question. These days, we are besieged by a plethora of diets, each claiming to have The Answer. There's Paleo, Keto, gluten-free, Atkins, Low Fat, Cabbage Soup, Mediterranean, Plant Paradox, juice cleansing, Military, and hundreds more diet plans. Every day, another book comes out with yet another diet—all filled with ideas conceived in the head and imposed on our bodies. No wonder my patients are confused, with all the contradictory yet convincing information out there. I confess, it *is* overwhelming!

I think Soraya's *core question* is: "What will help me be the healthiest I can be, so I can enjoy my life to the fullest and hopefully not get cancer, Alzheimer's, heart disease, diabetes or some other debilitating disease?"

Many of my patients have been told by doctors that they are risking heart disease by having high cholesterol, or that they have elevated blood sugar and will develop diabetes. They have been told that they need to lose weight, lower their cholesterol with drugs, and watch their blood sugar. The bottom line in the doctor's message is that they are in BIG DANGER. No wonder that they arrive in my office scared and anxious. They don't know what to do.

Soraya continued telling her story. "My brother fell dead of a heart attack at 52," she reported. "My sister suffered a stroke in her 40s. And my neighbor was just diagnosed with cancer. I don't want to end up the same way."

"There *is* room for hope," I reassured her. "Things *can* be improved. We have time to turn things around. But before I can advise you about what to eat," I went on, "I need to understand more thoroughly what is going on with you—to get the whole picture. Tell me about your life— your work and family life, and how you spend your day."

Then I sat back and listened, knowing that this process takes time. As a holistic physician, I expect my first appointment with a new patient to take about two hours. Slowly, we separate fact from fear. As I listen, I become better able to suggest ways that will support each patient to achieve her or his goal of optimal health.

"Do you have any medical problems?" I began.

"I've been overweight since the birth of my first child," she answered, "even though I tried Weight Watchers and various diets. My doctor is worried about my blood sugar, which has been a little high; and my cholesterol is also high."

"I noticed on your medical history form that you had some surgery," I prompted after Soraya had paused. "Can you tell me more about that?"

"I had a hysterectomy when I was 40 because I couldn't stop bleeding. My periods would last for weeks, and I was becoming anemic. The doctor tried putting me on birth-control pills, but they didn't help. I tried that new ablation treatment, but the bleeding came back after a few months. I was told the only thing was just to have my uterus taken out. Since then I've gained even more weight!"

"What about your family?" I probed further. "Are there other health conditions in the family that we should be aware of? You mentioned that your brother had a heart attack and your sister had a stroke."

"Both my parents developed diabetes when they got older. I don't know much about my grandparents, because they never went to doctors. My dad had a triple bypass in his 60s. My mom has some kind of thyroid condition, and so does her sister. Mom's really overweight and can barely get around. And my son has ADHD, but we're dealing with it."

"So there's some family history of problems with blood sugar, heart, and thyroid that you may have inherited a genetic predisposition to," I noted. (For more details about thyroid problems, see Chapter Nine: Fatigue and Recovery.)

"Yes." Soraya let out a big sigh. "And that's why I'm so worried. I want to avoid having those same problems. When I look in the mirror, I see my mother, and I'm afraid I'll end up like her! But I am so confused, I don't know what to do." Tears welled up in her eyes.

We sat together in silence for a moment, acknowledging the presence of her fear. Then I told her, "I think there's room for hope. But before I can advise you about what to eat, I need to know a little more about your current eating habits."

Soraya nodded her agreement and wiped her tears.

"Did you bring a food journal?" I asked. I request all new patients to record a week's food intake, as well as their mood and energy level, and to bring this record to their first appointment. Just looking at their journal tells me a lot. The very act of having to write down what one eats can create a new awareness, as well as make one feel more accountable; and the process may influence food choices from that time on. I am always grateful to the many patients who choose to record what they have eaten honestly, in hopes of getting insight and direction.

Soraya rummaged in her purse. "This wasn't a typical week," she apologized, as she handed me her notes. "I was especially busy, so I had to grab more meals on the run." Many patients tell me similar things as they hand me their food journals. Some say, "We were entertaining a lot this week," or "We were traveling, so I didn't eat my usual food."

But in reality, there *is* no "typical week." We hold an idealized notion of what we *want* to be eating, which may not look anything like what we actually *are* eating. Many people in today's too-busy world are eating lots of meals on the run, or are not even eating *meals* but just grabbing bites and bits of food all day. Many of us are not aware of the cumulative effect of our lifestyle choices on our dietary intake.

And then there are those patients who don't *bring* a food journal to their first appointment, which could be a measure of how overly busy their lives are. Some patients tell me honestly that they didn't feel good enough about their food choices to write them down. And sometimes they just plain forget to do it, or (if they did keep a food log) they forget to bring it with them. If they haven't brought a seven-day food log, I ask them to just relate what and when they ate during the previous twenty-four hours. It gives me some idea of what food choices they are making. I learn how often food is eaten on the run and how many meals a week are made at home. As we talk about food, I begin to understand the role that food plays in their life and what they already know about nutrition. (A sample of a Food Journal can be found in the Appendix, Chapter Three.)

"Tell me a little about food in your family when you were a child," I prompted Soraya. Our exposure to food as a child has a big influence on our food choices as an adult.

"My mother always worked," Soraya recalled, "so dinner was often something she could fix quickly when she got home. We usually had some meat and potatoes or rice, and canned or frozen vegetables. And there was always dessert. Mom always made sure there were cookies and snacks around for us, as well as for herself and dad."

"Did you eat together as a family very often?" I wanted to know.

"Oh yes, every night. Dinner was important to my parents and we had to be there."

Some of my patients grew up in homes where *no one* cooked—where frozen, pre-cooked food was delivered once a month, and the microwave was the main cooking method. These people rarely experienced the smell of onions cooking or of a chicken roasting in the oven. They were deprived of those important cooking smells, which activate the rhythms of our digestive system (as we learned in Chapter Two, on digestion). They also missed the opportunity to witness the process of bringing a meal to the table. The patients who got to participate and learned how to cook from a seasoned dedicated cook in the home were fortunate indeed.

Who Is Tending the Family Today?

When I started out in midwifery, I used to say that the family unit of health consisted of who ate out of the same refrigerator. Nowadays, it's more about who eats out of the same SUV. With both parents working or a single working parent heading the family, few families are cooking most of their meals at home. A lot of parents are spending every non-working hour ferrying kids to and from various afterschool activities or helping with homework, or both. Many people eat out or bring home prepared meals for half or more of their total meals each week.

Perhaps the biggest loss is that the role of *Hearth keeper* has been forgotten. The Greeks acknowledged this important role in the goddess Hestia. She is the one who keeps the home fires burning. That role—which, in the past, was traditionally filled by a mother, a grandmother, a maiden aunt, or perhaps a hired housekeeper—has been lost in the mad rush of modern daily life. Many houses are mere shells, holding space where people come and sleep but without that soulful quality that a true *home* provides. There are big beautiful kitchens that rarely emit the tantalizing smell of food cooking.

The Inconvenience of Convenience Foods

Life has become extremely hectic, with little free time for either the children or the adults. One effect of this fast pace has been the huge rise in fast-food restaurants and the drive-through, and the enormous availability of convenience foods. But the only thing *convenient* about "convenience foods" is that they require little preparation. They are often not fresh, usually not local, and rarely as nutritious as a freshly made home-cooked meal. (They also create more plastic-packaging waste.)

The really sad thing about the invasion of these convenience foods is that now there are generations who have grown up with little experience of home cooking. These folks have no sensual memory of the smell of food cooking in the kitchen, or of seeing food being prepared from scratch at home. When I meet these people in my consulting room, I am aware of this huge void in their toolbox of self-care. They have no personal legacy of home-cooked family favorites, nothing to build from to create their own repertoire of delicious and nutritious meals. For some, the experience of the whole family sitting down at the table and eating together was limited to Thanksgiving and maybe one or two other holidays. No wonder they don't like vegetables! They've never experienced freshly cooked, artfully seasoned fresh vegetables. In fact, many vegetables have never been experienced at all. These unfortunate people's knowledge of vegetables is limited to those that come in TV dinners or popped out of a can, microwaved and dumped on a plate: tasteless, limp, wholly unappetizing, and devoid of real nutritional value.

During my years of practice, I have tried several ways to help patients who wanted to improve their cooking skills. One of my secretaries was Greek and grew up in a kitchen full of people who cooked with joy and skill. Kathy loved cooking and good food, and her enthusiasm was contagious. She offered a series of cooking classes, and those patients who attended enjoyed it immensely. Together they learned to make spanakopita, lamb stew, baklava, and more. Each week they prepared and ate a complete meal the Greek way—with everyone in the kitchen laughing, talking, and participating.

Another innovation was Mothers Kitchen—a group program I started that was composed of new mothers who got together once a month to prepare food for their family. My original intention was to provide a way for the new mothers I was seeing in my practice to connect with other women who were also in various stages of mothering. To create a sort of village well, where women could gather and find support, information, and community in a natural, easeful way.

Each Mothers Kitchen gathering was focused on making a main dish, chosen beforehand by the group via email. Someone shopped for the ingredients, and another volunteered to lead the group. Each woman brought her pot or container, and left with a delicious dinner to cook and serve her family at home. We learned how to cut up a whole chicken; different ways to cut and cook fresh vegetables; how to spice, sauté, and marinate. While we worked, the women also had an opportunity to see other mothers managing their infants and toddlers. Sometimes grandmothers came to help with the toddlers. That was always a wonderful addition.

SOME NOURISHING TIPS

Cook your food at home.

❖

Smell the food while it's cooking—your senses will enjoy it and it will stimulate your appetite and digestive juices.

❖

Take time to enjoy eating what you have cooked.

❖

Give thanks—to yourself for cooking; for the food itself; and for those nourished by what you have cooked.

As we prepped, the mothers took nursing breaks, fed toddlers, gathered tips about gluten- and dairy-free breakfasts and snacks, and absorbed how other moms approached the challenges of balancing busy lives and many responsibilities. We laughed a lot and learned how to make stews, pesto, ginger ale, stir fry, and more. Eventually, Mothers Kitchen moved out of my kitchen and began to meet in the other women's homes. Later, a vegetarian Mothers' Kitchen started up as the idea spread. Some groups continued for years, until the children started school and life needs changed.

How Food Affects the Body

Just then Soraya spoke up: "I just want to know what is a good diet for me! I need help so I can make the right choices." Her voice sounded almost pleading.

"There is no simple answer to what you are asking," I explained. "We don't all wear a size-nine shoe; our feet are all different sizes. Likewise, our metabolism and genetic predispositions are unique and have unique nutritional needs. This is not about yet another diet. It's about healthy eating choices that will serve you for the rest of your life. We want to find the food choices that work best for *you*.

"So," I went on, "before we can talk about what food to choose, we need to understand a little more about how food affects your body. This understanding will help us to select foods that meet your body's unique needs." And I begin to explain in more detail.

Metabolic rate: "Your *metabolic rate* is like the thermostat setting for your body's furnace. If the thermostat is set low, your metabolism is low and slow. Many people feel cold, or chill easily, feel tired, or have low energy when their metabolism is slow. A slow metabolism means that you are burning fewer calories than someone with a faster metabolism." I could see Soraya's head nodding as I spoke.

I continued, "So if you eat more calories than your thermostat is set to burn, you will gain weight. People with a slow metabolism tell me things like, 'I can eat almost nothing for several days and never lose a pound, and I can gain weight just by eating normally.'"

"That's me *exactly*!" Soraya exclaimed, straightening up in her chair.

"There can be several reasons for having a slow metabolism," I continued. "A thyroid that is not functioning adequately can be a cause. Another possible cause occurs with people who have a *blood-sugar wobble*—a hyper-reactive pancreas that easily produces excessive amounts of insulin. Abnormally high insulin levels can slow metabolism and reduce the rate of calorie burning. At least 25 percent of the population has this problem. The fact that both your parents developed diabetes later in life makes it likely that you have inherited this blood-sugar wobble. Eating the Standard American (SAD) Diet can be a major contributor to raising insulin levels, which then slow down metabolism."

The Standard American Diet (SAD)

Sometimes, when I am in the supermarket or at the mall or an airport, I become saddened at the sight of so many overweight people. So many people are still in their 20s, 30s and 40s—relatively young—yet I can tell by the way they stand or walk that they are in pain and don't seem comfortable in their own bodies. They are overweight, and they look drained and strained.

Many Americans are suffering from *high-calorie malnutrition*. They are eating lots of calories, but their food does not contain enough of the essential nutrients that are needed to sustain a healthy body. I have heard that the average American consumes 22 teaspoons of sugar a day! That's a lot of kilocalories with little-to-no nutrient value—basically, empty calories. Refined flour, baked goods, pasta, and sodas are also essentially empty calories. People eat a lot of foods that fill them up but do not really provide much nourishment.

When I was a midwife in the 1970s, I was very concerned that the women in my care made good food choices, because an expectant mother who was well nourished and healthy was more likely to give birth easily with fewer complications.

Most of the women I cared for were planning a homebirth. Months before their due date, my assistant and I made a home visit to get a better sense of their family life, support systems, and quality of their nutrition. Somehow we always found an excuse to take a look in their refrigerators. If we found hot dogs, bologna, white bread, and American cheese, with few fruits or veggies, we knew that we had some work ahead of us to educate our client about nutrition. We knew that a woman on the SAD diet was unknowingly putting herself at higher risk for birth complications, such as a slow and ineffective labor, exhaustion, and excessive bleeding. She might also have a slower recovery and possible breastfeeding problems with milk supply, or mastitis, and a greater susceptibility to colds or other infections in the postpartum period.

The Standard American Diet is primarily composed of variations on milk and wheat. Breakfast is cereal with milk, often non- or low-fat milk; or a bagel and cream cheese; or a fruity yogurt with a pop tart or toast. Lunch is pizza, or mac-and-cheese, a cheese sandwich, or a cheeseburger and fries, maybe with a shake. And dinner might be more pizza, or spaghetti, lasagna, or another pasta-and-cheese concoction. Typically, *most* meals contain some form of milk and some form of wheat. Vegetables in the SAD world exist primarily as a salad (if at all), or something that appears at the Big Home-Cooked Meal of the Week, or maybe only at Thanksgiving or Christmas.

Most of the food in the SAD diet can be found in the middle of the supermarket, stacked in endless aisles with an almost eternal shelf life. The *living foods* that contain vital nutrients—the vegetables, fruit, milk products, meat, organ meats, seafood and eggs—are found around the edges of the supermarket.

Changing from SAD to SANE (Safe and Nutritious Eating)

Changing from the SAD way of eating is challenging. Indeed, the *current way of life* in America is challenging. We have lost the Hearth keeper. When all the adults in a family are needed to work an outside job, there is no one left to be a homemaker. No one is tending home base.

The recession that began in 2008 when the housing bubble burst has had some silver linings. Some young families have moved back into their parents' home. Many young people didn't have the resources to move out and live on their own. The multi-generational family, with an adult who stays at home, has become more common again. Once again, there may be someone who is home for children returning from school and adults returning from work. Someone who shops and cooks for the family. A new generation of Hearth keepers has been born out of necessity. A number of families in my practice live as a multi-generational unit, and most report that it works well for them.

Another positive development is the increased availability of fresh, local, non-processed food. Farmer's markets, CSAs (Community Sponsored Agriculture), and farm stores have multiplied exponentially. Today I see a new generation of people inspired to do the hard work of growing food and stewarding the land in good ways. Small local industries are sprouting up. One of my patients started a sauerkraut business, making organic, lacto-fermented sauerkraut on the farm, with her husband, her child and her parents all living together and working in the business. Another patient opened a business making organic skin-care products. Some have started raising free-range cows, pigs, sheep, chickens, and eggs, as well as organic vegetables.

We are starting to see a return of emphasis on *quality* versus *quantity*: quality of food, quality of life, quality of work, and quality of relationships. The bursting of the housing bubble and subsequent recession has stirred a re-examination of our values. Many now question values such as *more/bigger/newer/faster*, and consider that those qualities may not always be *better*. The impact and consequences of venerating those values is being reviewed in the light of a growing awareness of the fragility and preciousness of life on this beautiful planet.

Finding the Starting Point

As I shared all this with Soraya, I could see her taking it in. Her head was nodding, and a look of comprehension spread across her face. "I'm ready to make a change," she declared. "So where do I start?"

"Changing our routine is always a journey," I answered. "And, as the saying goes, 'The journey of a thousand miles begins with one step.' We begin by becoming aware of where we are. As psychologist Carl Rogers put it, 'The curious paradox is that, when I accept myself just as I am, then I can change.'"

I felt the need to say more. "We tend to judge ourselves pretty harshly. In reality, nothing is either all bad or all good. There is no one *right* way of eating any more than there is one right way to bring up your children, take care of a household, or spend your leisure time.

"Let's begin by letting go of any self-judgments you may have, and taking a look at what you are actually *choosing* to eat. If you know that some of your choices are not in your own best interest, then you are already ahead of the game."

Soraya nodded. "I know sometimes I choose foods that are not good for me, like cake or candy. Then I feel bad that I did it." Her voice dropped, and she frowned at the floor.

I reassured her, "This is not about shaming or blaming. It's about finding what food choices make you feel good, and that also will help you avoid some of the health problems that run in your family."

Together, we reviewed the seven-day food log that she had brought with her. It seemed that her breakfast was often coffee with non-dairy creamer, and a protein shake. Snacks during the day were Ritz crackers or a granola bar (gluten-free), or a waffle, which were eaten on the run. Dinner might be take-out or frozen food, or something eaten at a restaurant. Sometimes it was a microwaved hot dog and a sweet potato.

The first red flag on her list was the creamer. What's sold as "creamer" is usually a non-dairy product consisting of various chemicals designed to give a white coloring, sweetness, and creamy texture. These ingredients contain nothing of nutritional value, and the chemicals are difficult for the human digestive system to handle.

I suggested, "Well, for starters, you could use heavy cream or half-and-half in your coffee, instead of artificial creamer."

"Wow! Real cream?" She seemed delighted with the idea. But there was a doubting tone in her voice.

"Why not? It's not only healthier, but it tastes a great deal better!"

"No problem there, I can make that change," Soraya reassured me.

"Next, let's figure out how many of these foods are *simple carbohydrates*. Simple carbohydrates break down into blood sugar very quickly and can stimulate high insulin levels, which lower your metabolism. We want to choose foods that *raise* your metabolism, not lower it."

I explained further, "Simple carbohydrates would include bread, crackers, pasta, chips, candy, cakes, cookies, soda—and also potatoes, fruit juices, bananas (surprise!), and cereals." And I handed Sophia a highlighter to mark the foods in her journal that were simple carbohydrates.

When I do this exercise together with my patients, many are surprised at what they learn. Because I ask them to chart their mood and energy level as well as what they eat, they begin to see a connection between their food intake and its effect. Often meals missed or meals high in simple carbohydrates precede periods of fatigue or slowed mental functioning.

Once we had reviewed what she had been eating, I told her, "Now that we know our starting point, we can begin our journey. The next step is to decide what we will change."

Deciding What to Change in Your Diet

And here's where my knowing more about the kind of person Soraya is can help me to help her. The kind of person who dives into the deep end of the pool and starts swimming is a very different person than the one who would rather sit on the edge of the pool and dangle her feet in the water a while. And they both are different from the one who slowly but steadily takes the steps, starting at the shallow end, and then finally pushes off and swims.

So I said to her, "You may want to make big changes all at once, or take gradual smaller steps. If you like the big-change idea—if changing a lot of things all at once about the way you eat works better for you—then I would suggest that you consider removing about 80 percent of the starchy or simple carbohydrate foods that you currently eat." I paused to see her response.

WHICH WAY OF MAKING CHANGES FITS YOU? (A SWIMMING ANALOGY):

Big, instant change — diving into the deep end and swimming right away

Slow change — sitting at the pool's edge and dangling your feet until you're ready

Steady change — starting at the shallow end, then slowly, steadily, going deeper

Reducing Carbohydrates

Farmers have long known that if you want to fatten an animal up before slaughter, you feed it carbohydrates, such as grains. I have a clipping from a local farming magazine of a bunch of cows drinking from one of those huge aluminum water-tanks, with two farmers looking on. But the liquid in the tank is not water—it's soda! The caption under the picture states that the farmer had made an arrangement with a local soda company to get their excess. It mentions that the farmer finds this alternative food source (sugar) very effective in speeding up weight gain in his cows. That's what carbohydrates do best: put on the weight.

Soraya asked me, "Should I just cut out *all* the carbohydrates?" She was obviously ready to plunge into the deep end of the pool.

I smiled. "Removing simple carbohydrates from your diet alone is not enough to shift your metabolism, unless you also *add* good saturated fats to your diet. Furthermore, it's very important that you eat a good portion of protein and fat every four hours. This helps maintain a higher metabolic rate, and prevents hunger pangs.

"It is not necessary to remove all carbohydrates," I advised her. "Let's begin by eliminating all *processed* carbohydrates, such as products that contain flour and added sugars. This includes products labeled 'whole-grain.' Although originally whole-grain, in its current form as finely ground flour it has lost much of its nutritional value and has become a simple carbohydrate."

"So I can keep *some* carbohydrates in my diet?" Soraya asked.

"Just as no one diet suits all people because each person is different and unique," I told her, "not all carbohydrates are equal. Some carbohydrates—such as sweet potatoes, beans, and whole-grains—are very important to provide enough calories for children and athletically active adults. Grains, in their whole-grain (not pulverized) form are complex carbohydrates and do not stimulate an insulin burst in the same way that flour does. Whole grains break down into blood sugar more slowly than flour products. And it's important to have plenty of good saturated fats."

Good Saturated Fats

Soraya suddenly looked puzzled. "What are *good* saturated fats?"

"We have been told that saturated fats are the *bad* fats, right? We've been told wrong. There are many *good* saturated fats. Good saturated fat comes from healthy, pasture-raised animals that have not been given antibiotics, steroids, or other hormones, and preferably whose diet is also GMO-free and organic. Good saturated fats include the animal-based fats like lard, suet (beef fat), chicken fat, duck fat, fish oil, butter, and cream, as well as coconut and palm oil. It's important that they are organic or come from pastured animals."

Soraya's jaw had dropped and she was listening intently.

I continued, "Another important source of good saturated fat comes from fish, which contains important omega-3 fat. Most people's diets are deficient in omega-3 fat, which is plentiful in fish oil. Another little-known fact is that the fat in eggs and chickens that are pasture-raised has significantly more omega-3 fat than eggs or chickens from factory-farmed animals. There's been a lot in the news about the importance of omega-3 fatty acids and their contribution to reducing inflammation. A number of studies show a correlation between the low levels of omega-3 fatty acids and higher incidence of heart disease, stroke, and Alzheimer's, among other diseases. The pharmaceutical industry is trying to capitalize on this information and recently came out with a prescription omega-3 for doctors to prescribe."

A SANE DIET INCLUDES GOOD SATURATED FATS:

Lard
Beef fat (suet)
Chicken fat
Duck Fat
Fish Oil
Butter
Cream
Coconut Oil
Palm Oil

Soraya's brow furrowed. She burst in, "What's wrong with using vegetable oils?"

I explained, "Vegetable oils are polyunsaturated oils. Chemically, they are less stable than saturated fats, and can become rancid much more easily. Sometimes chemicals such as BHT are added to products containing polyunsaturated oils to prevent rancidity. BHT and other chemical antioxidants have been linked to cancer in rats, and actually are banned in some countries, such as England. In addition, unless the vegetable oils are organic they will contain pesticide residues, which are carcinogenic."

"But I thought saturated fats were the Bad Ones?" Soraya looked confused.

I nodded. "*Good* saturated fats need to be distinguished from *bad* saturated fats. One of the characteristics of saturated fats is that they become solid at cooler temperatures. A polyunsaturated oil (such as safflower, cottonseed, soy, or corn oil) can be artificially hydrogenated and become a saturated fat (such as Crisco or margarine.) These *artificially hydrogenated* oils are called *trans* fats, and they *are* the bad guys. They form chemical bonds that are different from those saturated fats that occur naturally in nature. Polyunsaturated fats are known to increase the number of free radicals in the body. The increase in free radicals has long been associated with cancer. Trans fats are also known to cause cancer.

"So stay away from *trans* fats as well as polyunsaturated fats," I concluded. "It helps that manufacturers recently have been required to label any trans fats."

Many shelf-hardy foods (cookies, crackers, chips, and the like) have artificially hydrogenated (trans) fats listed in their ingredients. The trans fats will keep them crisp on the shelf for much longer than is the case for a naturally saturated fat. Many peanut butters contain artificially hydrogenated oils, which give them a creamy texture and prevent oil from gathering at the top of the jar. *That's another good reason to read the Ingredients list on the product label.*

A diet developed by Johns Hopkins has 80 percent of its caloric intake coming from saturated fats. Named the *Ketogenic Diet*, Hopkins created it as treatment for babies and children who were having seizures all the time, and whose epilepsy could not be controlled by medication. The Ketogenic Diet substantially reduced the children's seizure activity, and these same children grew and thrived.

Back in the 1950s, Dr. Baroda Barnes observed beneficial results in his patients who removed high-carbohydrate foods from their diet and added good saturated fats to all their meals. He was way ahead of Dr. Atkins, who made the same discovery years later. In fact, as far back as 1892, doctors have been documenting successful weight loss and maintenance with patients on low-carbohydrate, high-fat diets. I have met many people who told me that the only way they successfully lost weight was when they went on the "Atkins diet"—meaning a diet low in carbohydrates and high in fat content.

Making a Lifestyle Shift

At the end of our long discussion, Soraya returned to her original question: "So, what diet *should* I be on?"

"The real answer," I said, "is to *stop thinking in short-term solutions!* Instead of viewing what you eat as a 'diet,' which implies a temporary 'fix,' start to see your choices as laying the foundation for a lifetime of health. Use nourishing yourself as another way to express *self-care* and *self-loving*.

Your goal is to develop a new way of eating that includes food choices that will be yours for the rest of your life.

"Not another diet. Not another temporary fix. If your goal is to get healthy and *stay* healthy, to feel good and stay in the best shape, you don't want yet another diet. *What will really serve you best is to find your personal food melody that you can dance to for the rest of your life.*"

> *Use nourishing yourself as another way to express self-care and self-loving. Your goal is to develop a new way of eating that includes food choices that will be yours for the rest of your life.*

Soraya's head was nodding vigorously in agreement, so I went on: "What we are really talking about is making a *lifestyle shift*. It's about you, as an adult in the driver's seat, choosing to do it differently—choosing to make different food choices. The really good news is that once you are over the hump of making changes and have settled into your new pattern and choices, you will feel good. And *feeling good is its own reward*. What's more, when you feel good, you are motivated to *continue* to feel good; and the desire for those empty-calorie, high-carbohydrate foods fades away. The sugar cravings usually are gone after a week."

"Wow," she sighed. "Well, I think I've eaten enough donuts to last me the rest of my life!"

"Just remember," I said, "the key to success is to make sure that you are eating adequate portions of protein and fats *every four hours*. Protein and fats break down very slowly into blood sugar. They provide a steady input of glucose into our bodies over three to four hours, which keeps our insulin levels steady and our metabolism humming at a good rate. However, it is important to replenish the fuel at regular intervals to ensure that the furnace continues to burn at its new level. You want to avoid the drastic ups and downs of blood sugar."

"I'm ready to make a change!" Soraya declared, straightening up in her chair. "I just need help figuring out what to eat, now."

So together, Soraya and I made up a meal plan for her that included protein and fat every four hours. Soraya picked the foods she liked, and I suggested other protein- and fat-rich food, such as nut butters (containing only nuts and salt); sardines; hummus or guacamole, eaten with veggies; numerous egg dishes, including deviled eggs and egg salad; and sugar-free and nitrate-free bacon, natural salami, pâté, terrines, and sausage.

"It's important to have a hearty snack of protein and fat about four hours after you eat lunch," I advised. "That will help you arrive home in the evening not famished and less tempted to snack on high-carb snack foods while you get ready for dinner."

Before Soraya left, I had some parting words: "Before you start on your new food plan, take some time to get the food you will need home and ready. Don't forget to eat plenty of organic butter. And if you run into any problems or have any questions, please call me. Remember, I'm on your support team now."

Her smile stretched across her face. "My husband's going to love this! Bacon and eggs for breakfast! Real butter! I can't wait to tell him."

We made plans to follow up in six weeks and see how things were going for her at that point.

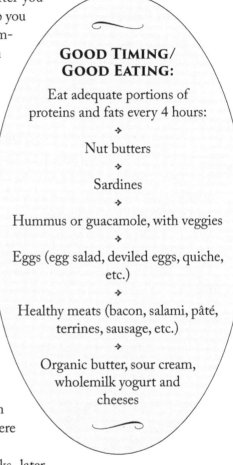

GOOD TIMING/ GOOD EATING:

Eat adequate portions of proteins and fats every 4 hours:

Nut butters

Sardines

Hummus or guacamole, with veggies

Eggs (egg salad, deviled eggs, quiche, etc.)

Healthy meats (bacon, salami, pâté, terrines, sausage, etc.)

Organic butter, sour cream, wholemilk yogurt and cheeses

At our appointment six weeks later, Soraya reported that she had taken some time to get ready before changing her eating habits. For about four weeks, she had been eating fewer carbohydrates and more fat. She already noticed a change in how her clothes fit and she felt that her energy had improved significantly. She reported that her husband had also lost weight, and both of them were enjoying eating more home-cooked meals. She was pleased with the developments, and so was I.

ANSWERS TO COMMON QUESTIONS ABOUT HEALTHY FOOD CHOICES

The following are questions that I am frequently asked when food choices are discussed.

"How Do I Find Time to Make *All This Food?"*

One problem is that the amount of time that people need to spend on food preparation increases as they begin to prepare meals from whole foods, rather than buying convenience foods. This means that time spent doing something else has to decrease—maybe watching less TV, or spending less time on Facebook.

If you are motivated, you will find a way to make shopping and cooking a priority. Perhaps these activities will become part of what you and your family do together, or will be time when you and your partner can unwind after work and catch up with each other. Put on some music you love. Listen to that audio book you've been wanting to read while you cook. Fill your kitchen with pleasantness and comfort to make it a juicy, nourishing place. Let these times feed your spirit as well as your body.

As you make your food, invest these food-preparation times with thoughts of goodness and all the wellbeing you are giving yourself. No kidding. This is *"me time"*—time given to support and love oneself, not another punitive regimen that you are enduring only until some destination point is reached and then quickly shrugged off. These activities of self-care and -tending are vital in building your new life—just as vital to your journey as every other step you take. Eventually, they become your reliable companions on the journey to health and wellness. *Remember: it takes 25 days of doing something differently before it becomes a habit.*

Sally Fallon, the author of *Nourishing Traditions*, suggests that making your own salad dressing using olive oil is a very important first food to learn. Mix together 3 parts oil and 1 part vinegar. Add salt and pepper to taste, and use spices if you want, such as thyme, basil, or oregano (however, plain is also delicious). Vinegars such as balsamic, rice, apple cider, or another vinegar are all good options, and each adds its own particular nuance. Shake or stir well before using. This dressing can be made ahead in large quantities and will stay well on the counter for at least a week, and weeks in the refrigerator.

"Should I Avoid Salt?"

The short answer is NO. Dr. Weston Price, a dentist, spent over 20 years researching the diets of people with perfect dental health (no cavities or gum disease). These people were all eating food that was prepared in the same way as their grandmothers' grandmothers had done. He called these people's diet "traditional," to contrast them with the diets of people who had added modern processed foods. He found that salt was used in all the traditional diets around the world.

The oldest trade routes in the world that we know about were used to trade salt. Animals will walk miles to natural salt licks. Adequate salt is key to health, as the ancients knew and animals instinctively know.

Although there has been a widespread myth that salt is bad for you, there is little evidence to support that myth. Salt intake has been linked to high blood pressure; however, in those studies that looked at total intake of salt and found a correlation to blood pressure, the source of the salt was not clarified.

What this means is that it makes a lot of difference whether the salt in the total count came from processed foods, canned foods, or just sea salt added to cooking or on the table. Why? Because there could be many other chemicals in processed foods besides salt that contribute to raising blood pressure. Other than the few people who swell when they eat salt, everyone else should be salting their food to satisfy their palates. The salt shaker needs to be back on the table. And, ideally, use unprocessed, unbleached sea salt.

"How Important Are Vegetables?"

Vegetables are our friends. They come naturally full of fiber, not to mention vitamins and minerals. Remember what I said at the start of this chapter about how recent nutrition news is all about getting enough fiber in our diets? It's true—we *do* need fiber in our diet. It helps bulk up our stools, so that our bowels work more efficiently and effectively.

Vegetables are a perfect source of fiber. If we are eating five servings of vegetables a day (not the starchy ones), we are getting enough fiber. A "serving" consists of one cup of raw veggies or one-half cup of cooked vegetables.

However, a fiber bar is not the equivalent of a cup or two of broccoli. The food industry has capitalized on the attention given to fiber and made a fortune adding grain chaff to candy bars and calling them "fiber bars." People are buying them hand over fist, thinking that they are making a healthier choice than with their old candy bars. Sadly, their new choices of breakfast bars, fiber bars, or protein bars are little improvement. These bars are usually high in sugars and carbohydrates, and are not adequate replacements for a real meal of protein, vegetables, and good fat.

"But What If I Don't Like Vegetables?"

Over the years of working with people on their food choices, I have discovered that many of them grew up *hating* vegetables. Perhaps vegetables were never served at their childhood home. Or if they were, they were accompanied with remarks like, "You're not leaving the table until you've finished your vegetables." Often, those vegetables were canned or frozen and simply heated up and dumped on the plate. They were not very tasty, to say the least. A lot of people grew up with the spoken or unspoken message that vegetables were an unpleasant business, to be endured with resignation or resisted at all costs.

These same folks have usually had a very limited exposure to the World of Vegetables. I have known many people whose experience with vegetables was limited to broccoli, green beans, carrots, peas, lima beans and corn. Yes, those *are* vegetables. However, corn, lima beans, and peas are primarily starchy carbohydrates. They are low in fiber and should be limited in your new regimen.

But there is good news! For those infrequent flyers to the World of Vegetables, there's a whole tantalizing *world* of vegetables you are about to discover.

If I'm working with children who have been vegetable-avoidant, I suggest that they begin to keep a food journal titled, "New Vegetables I Have Met." They are instructed to pick one new vegetable each week that they haven't ever tried before. During that week, they are to try eating it prepared a few different ways. They can eat it steamed, plain with lots of butter, and salted to taste. Another day, they might have it roasted in coconut oil, or sautéed in butter or bacon fat, or with sausage and onions. They can try putting it in stews, barbequing it, or grating it raw and having it in a salad. (Grated beets and turnips are amazingly delicious in a salad.) Some adults have found that keeping a "New Vegetables I Have Met" journal is a helpful tool for them, too.

> *Vegetables are not limited to what you may have been served as a child. There are veggies you may not yet have tasted (or known ones you may develop a taste for); and they can be prepared in an almost infinite (and delicious!) number of ways.*

There's a whole host of amazing vegetables available in today's savvy supermarkets. And if you go to a supermarket that caters to Hispanic or Oriental folks, you'll discover an expanded array of vegetables that your local supermarket may not carry. Your explorations in the World of Vegetables can become quite exciting.

When these veggie-phobic children return to my office, together we review their Vegetable Journal and the discoveries they have made. Many times I notice that their attitude towards vegetables has changed. They have been helping their parents with preparing these new foods, and have enjoyed learning new skills such as using a knife or a grater; stirring things on the stove; or looking up recipes on the Internet. Obviously, a child is going to need an adult who is onboard with this plan and willing to assist. Many times, the journey of discovery has been beneficial for the adults in the family as well as the child.

So now we have added new skills and experiences to our food adventure. Our horizons are expanding. My hope is that they continue to expand over time. If you are fortunate and live where local seasonal vegetables are available, you will discover the world of difference in taste and texture between a freshly picked vegetable that has traveled less than 50 miles to market compared to one that's traveled 3,000 miles or more. Most of us are already aware of the difference in flavor between locally grown tomatoes just in from the garden and those hauled in from a distance or fetched from cold storage. No comparison, right?

Some people join a Community Sponsored Agriculture group, or CSA. With a CSA, you sign on with a farm in the spring and give them money then so they can use it to buy seeds and other equipment that they will need to grow the produce. In return, you are guaranteed an agreed-upon amount of produce that the farm produces from May through October or November. The details vary, depending on the location of the farm. Some grow food all year round (in poly tunnels or outside). Some CSAs deliver their produce to your home or a central distribution point. Others have you pick it up on the farm. Some have you pick it yourself, or work in partial exchange for the cost. Some CSAs also have eggs, chicken, beef, lamb, and dairy products for sale. Just remember: not all CSAs grow food organically, so choose one that does.

"Why Is Organic So Important?"

Many of the pesticides used on crops today contain chemicals that have estrogenic effects in our body called xeno-estrogens. When we eat foods that have been treated with these pesticides, our body's estrogen receptors pick them up in addition to our naturally occurring estrogen. This gives us excess estrogen, more than our bodies would normally make. Is it enough to make a difference? You bet.

I live in Maryland, near the Potomac River. About every five years, I see an article in the local newspaper about fish caught in the Potomac that have hermaphroditic features. These fish are males who also have developed female characteristics. The cause is the xeno-estrogens in the pesticide runoff from farmland into tributaries to the river. And it's not just the Potomac; the same pesticide residues are in many of our rivers today. In the Florida Everglades, alligators are developing micropenises, preventing them from copulating and producing young.

Ever wonder where "man boobs" come from? It's not just from being overweight; a lot of cities near me get their city water from the Potomac River, including Washington, D.C. The effect of pesticide residues in our foods has also become a major contributor to premature puberty. It may also be contributing to the lower sperm-count levels that are now considered normal in the U.S. When we eat meat from animals that were given grains grown with pesticides, the pesticide residues pass on to us.

Many pesticides contain heavy metals and other chemicals that affect and alter our bodies. Some chemicals affect our neurological function. Some are known to be carcinogenic; that is, they stimulate conditions that support the growth of cancer.

A particular subgroup of herbicides, called *neonicotinoids*, has been proven to be harmful to bees and a major cause of colony collapse, which has decimated the honeybee population. Some countries have banned the use of neonicotinoids, and their bee colonies are recovering. We need the bees for more than honey. They are major contributors to the health of the planet.

I understand that weeds (a frequent reason for pesticide use) are a problem for the farmer. Farmers have been struggling with weeds since the beginning of farming. Many farmers today have invested a lot of their money in expensive equipment and seed that is dependent on pesticide and herbicide use to control the pests and weeds. Farming has always been a hard business to make a profit from, because of so many variables—weather, market prices, disease, and other factors. The agrichemical business, in contrast, is making a lot of money. There's big money to be made in chemicals and genetically engineered seed.

However, there is a better, more sustainable way to farm. Many farmers have switched over to using organic methods of weed control and alternative soil-enrichment techniques, with good success. There are other benefits for the farmers as well; a study of organic farmers in Sweden found that their sperm counts were considerably higher compared to those of other males in their age group.

Maybe what we need to do is educate the consumer. The fruit or vegetable with a spot or imperfection is not only still quite edible but may even be desirable. I have noticed that the bugs and birds always pick the *sweetest* fruit to nibble on, not necessarily the prettiest. Organically grown fruits and vegetables are generally much more flavorful, as well as being better for you.

"Are Meat and Dairy Products Healthy?"

The old adage, "garbage in, garbage out," is certainly true for the animal products we eat. Today's commercially raised beef lives its life in a crowded feedlot, forced to eat whatever is put in the trough, which—up until the

Mad Cow Disease outbreak in the 1990s—included ground-up carcasses of cattle and other dead ruminants. These animals are forced to eat things that they would never choose over a pasture of grass, if given the choice. That feedlot animal, caged chicken, or penned hog has also been given antibiotics and steroids, which serve the two-fold purpose of both hastening weight gain and keeping the animal alive long enough to be slaughtered. It's not a big stretch to compare their life to a concentration camp or prison camp existence. And all those chemicals, as well as the adrenalin stirred up by the stress they are under, ends up in the meat.

I can understand why so many young people become vegetarians and vegans after learning what goes on inside America's commercial meat, egg, and dairy production. Even the fish that are farmed are fed soy and corn—food that no fish in the wild would be eating or even recognize as food.

The quality of the animal products—milk products, eggs, and meat—is very much related to the quality of the animals' lives. Chickens that are free-ranging and eating bugs, grass, and whatever else they find have a higher content of Omega-3 fat in their eggs than do caged birds that are fed a factory diet. Grass-fed beef has more minerals and more Vitamins A, D, E, and K.

"How did saturated fat and cholesterol become linked to heart disease?" In 1950, doctors began to notice a drastic rise in heart disease, which had suddenly become the number-one cause of death in the United States. Studies were begun to try to determine what factors were creating this increasingly worrisome health problem. In the 1960s, doctors doing autopsies on young American soldiers killed in the Vietnam War were shocked to see atherosclerotic plaque already built up and narrowing their arteries. These were men considered to be in the physical prime of their lives. Clearly, atherosclerotic plaque and hardening of the arteries was not just the result of ageing, as had been previously assumed.

Scientists began looking for the cause for the increase in heart disease, and a number of different theories emerged. One group thought that the amount of fat in the diet was a key factor. Another group felt that it was the ratio of saturated to unsaturated fat that was important, while another thought the percentage of calories from simple carbohydrates and sugars was most influential. Yet another group favored the theory that red meat was at the root of the problem. None of the studies was sufficiently robust, scientifically speaking, to rule in or rule out any one of these theories.

One scientist, Dr. Ancel Keys, a biologist and physiologist, became a key influencer in advancing the theory that dietary fat intake was directly linked to cholesterol levels which were, in turn, linked to heart disease. His most frequently cited study of seven countries looked at diet and the correlation to heart disease. The study showed a correlation between the amount of animal products (which contain saturated fats) in the diet, and the incidence of heart disease in the population. However, *correlation* does not prove *causation*. In fact, clinical trials have never been able to prove causation between the amount of saturated fats in the diet and heart disease. Many different countries have been studied since then, and there have been a number of other scientists who found evidence that contradicts Keys' conclusions.

Keys, however, was well connected and had the ear of the American Heart Association and the National Institute of Health. Even though his study was small and his hypothesis had not been tested for validity with any clinical trials, the idea that a simple cause for heart disease could be identified was too tempting to ignore. Keys felt people should restrict their intake of animal products because they contained saturated fats. The low-fat diet, with low *saturated fats* in particular, became the last word in heart health, and continues to be the accepted truth for most doctors today as well as the general public.

In 1980, the USDA food pyramid recommended that the majority of calories come from carbohydrates, while animal products—such as meat, milk, and eggs—should make up only a minor part of a person's diet. These dietary recommendations have been taken as gospel for an entire population of men, women, and even children in the United States. School breakfast and lunch programs have followed these guidelines. Hospital dieticians and diabetes counselors have all followed these same guidelines. This, despite the fact that many studies—including the longest-running study, the Framingham Heart Study—have *failed to confirm any correlation* between dietary saturated-fat intake and cholesterol levels *or* heart disease.

The Framingham Heart Study began in 1948 to study some 5,000 middle-aged men and women who lived in the small town of Framingham, Massachusetts. Every factor that researchers thought might be important in determining heart disease was surveyed at regular intervals. Six years into the study, research seemed to point to a correlation between high total cholesterol and heart disease. However, thirty years later, when there was much more data available, the predictive power of cholesterol levels as a measure of heart disease failed to prove true. In the Framingham Study, *half* the people who had heart attacks had cholesterol levels below 220 mg/dL, which was then considered the top normal number. Based on the Framingham Study, it would be hard to use cholesterol levels as a predictor of heart disease. The study also found absolutely no correlation between cholesterol levels and egg consumption, another myth that has had a hard time dying.

We can be encouraged by the fact that in 2016, the U.S. government issued dietary guidelines that no longer called for a limit on cholesterol. They also mentioned that three to five cups of coffee a day is not a problem for heart health.

For a more complete understanding of the low-fat versus low-carbohydrate diet controversy that has been on-going for the past sixty years, I recommend reading *The Big Fat Lie*, by Nina Teicholz. The book contains a wealth of details regarding the various epidemiological studies and clinical trials of dietary effects on heart disease that have been conducted over the years, as well as anecdotal evidence. The book goes a long way towards dispelling the myth that fat is bad for health.

"Is there a connection between red meat and heart disease?" Since the 1980 USDA food-pyramid guidelines and the AHA recommendations to avoid saturated fats, Americans have dutifully decreased their consumption of red meat. What has significantly *increased* is the consumption of cereals, pasta, and breads. What has *also* significantly increased is the incidence of obesity, diabetes, and heart disease, as well as children diagnosed on the autism spectrum.

It is only since 2000 that the data from large-scale clinical trials of low-fat and low-carbohydrate diets has been seeping into public awareness. These large studies failed to show any correlation between a low-fat diet and heart health. On the contrary, they demonstrated a *significant decrease* in obesity, diabetes, and heart disease to be correlated with diets containing higher percentages of animal products, including high saturated-fat levels combined with a low-carbohydrate intake.

Some studies showed that the men with the highest red-meat consumption also had the highest incidence of heart disease. However, the men in those studies also had the highest incidence of smoking and the least amount of exercise. Which of these factors—red meat, smoking, or lack of exercise—was most influential in promoting their heart disease is not clear. We do know that exercise and non-smoking are beneficial to the heart. Whether the health effect of red meat is primarily due to the presence of saturated fat, the health of the animal as a whole, or other factors in the meat has not been clarified yet.

"Does the quality of meat matter?" The answer that makes good health-sense is to eat the meat of healthy animals. There is some evidence already available that a healthier option for eating animal products is to buy pasture-raised, grass-fed beef, buffalo, and lamb, as well as free-range chicken, pork, and turkey. Choose meat from animals that have been raised in a humane and healthy environment, eating their traditional diet.

And it is important to eat the fat that comes with the meat. Eat the skin on the chicken. When I first ate organic, chemical-free, free-range chicken, I was amazed to find that it tasted like the chicken I remember from my childhood—full of real flavor and moistness (unlike the boneless, skinless chicken breasts that have become ubiquitous today).

It also makes sense to eat animal products such as eggs, butter, cheese, and other full-fat milk products from free-range animals fed organically. The fat of animals that are certified as "organic" will not contain pesticide residues, hormones, and steroids. *That* fat is *good* fat! So eat the fat on the free-range organic pork chop, and the skin on the organic chicken, and *all* the delicious fatty parts that human beings have known for eons are the tastiest and most satisfying. Eat without guilt, because eating fat does not make you fat. Eat without fear, because that fat will help raise your metabolism and give you a sense of satiety and wellbeing.

"How do I find organic, free-range animal products?" The Weston A. Price Foundation has done a wonderful job of collecting data about which farms sell organic produce, raw-milk products, and pasture-raised animal products. Go to their website (listed in the Appendix under Chapter Three: Nutrition) and look for the Chapter Leader nearest to you. That person has volunteered to keep an updated list of farms and food sources local to their area that sell organic and pasture-raised animal products. These Chapter Leaders serve as a worldwide grassroots network. They provide information to help consumers make good food choices as well as to support local farmers.

"But isn't organic expensive?" Yes, organic food *is* more expensive. Part of the reason is that it takes longer for a pastured, organic animal to grow than one fed chemicals and hormones to "beef it up" quickly. And producing vegetables and fruit organically also requires more labor.

Organic food *is* more expensive; however, we want our farmers to be paid a living wage so that they can continue to survive as organic farmers. One way to reduce the cost of organic produce, meat, and animal products is to buy directly from the farmer.

> **ORGANIC MEAT:**
>
> Pasture-raised, grass-fed meat is healthier and more humane.
>
> Eat the fat—it's good for you and delicious!
>
> The products of healthy pasture-raised animals (eggs, butter, cream, cheese, milk, etc.) are chemical-free and healthy.

Doing so means that you can cut out the middleman costs. For example, I buy my chicken and pork from a friend who raises a small number of chickens and pigs each year; I buy my beef and lamb from another farmer down the road who feeds her cows and sheep on pasture grass. What's the benefit? I know where my food is coming from, and I see for myself how these farmers treat their animals. What's more, grass-fed meat from healthy animals is so delicious! It seems to me that health and pleasure walk hand- in-hand on this journey of wellbeing.

> *Health and pleasure walk hand-in-hand on the journey of wellbeing.*

"Do I Need to Take Vitamins?"

"Should I take vitamins?" is the million-dollar question! (I have probably been asked this a million times.)

My answer is neither YES nor NO, but *"It depends."*

It depends on many different things. Most importantly, it depends on how you *feel or think* about taking vitamins. If you find yourself forgetting to take them more than remembering, take a look at that. Ask yourself,

"Am I also forgetting other aspects of self-care?" If you are too busy to stop and take vitamins, what in your life *are* you making time for, and how is that working for you?

Opinions on whether taking vitamins is helpful range from total enthusiasm to complete skepticism. The term "vitamins" is used to include all additional supplements, including herbs. Some people think that if they eat a well-balanced diet, they should be getting all the vitamins and minerals they need. Others feel that taking their supplements is what is keeping them healthy.

Who is correct? Remember, we are talking about the mind-body-spirit, not just the body. I tend to think that each person's point of view has a grain of truth in it—for them. Many studies have been done to determine whether this or that supplement is effective, and most of the time the results are less than decisive. My interpretation? This is another case in which the whole truth is not so easy to decipher, and each person's personal experience with supplements is key.

I think that a person's attitudes, both conscious and unconscious, make a huge difference in whether or not vitamins or other nutritional supplements will be helpful. If the care and regimentation of taking vitamins on a daily basis gives you a sense that you are doing something good for yourself—that is, that it's an act of self-love, a moment of "me time" that feels positive, hopeful, supportive, nurturing, and loving—then I think that taking vitamins is a good thing for you.

If, on the other hand, you are taking vitamins thinking, "I am so sick of taking these damn things!" it may be time to take a break and stop taking them for a while. If you are taking them to avoid a confrontation or a nagging reminder, then perhaps you have relinquished responsibility for your wellbeing to someone else (e.g., a spouse, child, friend). Or maybe vitamins have become just another piece of ammunition in an on-going battle with that person, and it's time to acknowledge the core issues in the conflict.

My point is: if you are not self-motivated to support your health in this way, then I don't think taking vitamins is a good thing for you at this time. Continually re-engaging in the negative thoughts and emotions that have become associated with taking vitamins may perhaps do more harm than good.

So think about whether you want to take vitamins, and why. Then create a program that works for you. Most of us have a hard time remembering to take *anything* two or three times a day, so make a schedule that works for you and meets your needs.

If someone has any underlying problems in digestion, then adding any vitamins or other supplements makes no sense. It is, in fact, a waste of time and money; the first thing to work on, in those circumstances, is restoring good digestion.

I ask my patients to bring all the supplements they are currently taking to our first appointment. The variety of amounts and approaches is striking. Some people bring in a few bottles. Others bring boxes and bags full, having rounded up everything in the house and wanting my opinion on whether they should take them, and which ones. Still others bring in impressive spreadsheets listing each supplement, as well as how often they take them. As for timing, some people take their supplements occasionally, when they remember. For others, it is a cornerstone of their self-care rituals. And as for purchasing, some have picked up their supplements at the big-box store, while others have carefully shopped online or at the health-food store.

"Do vitamins vary in quality?" In reviewing all these products, I have noted that the quality of vitamins and other supplements does vary widely. Those from the supermarket or big-box store tend to have a lot of artificial colors and flavors, as well as added sugars and other products. Some contain fillers, such as polypropylene glycol, magnesium stearate, and other chemicals that are used in the manufacturing process but are not desirable ingredients.

In general, I recommend avoiding supplements with *any* added artificial ingredients. Read the fine print on the labels, and choose ones that are free of gluten, soy, zein (a corn protein), corn, and dairy.

There is limited government oversight on vitamin and other nutritional supplements in the United States. For example, no one is checking to see if the product labeled Vitamin D3 actually *contains* Vitamin D3. So there is no guarantee that the label lists the *actual* ingredients in the bottle. The FDA's role regarding over-the-counter vitamins and supplements is primarily to review the labels and make sure that no medical claims are made about the products. The label on Vitamin D3 cannot claim to improve bone density or cure cancer, for example. To upgrade their reputation, some of the vitamin companies (for example, Thorne) have established their own quality-assurance programs to ensure a high standard of accountability.

"Is it possible to take too many vitamins?" There are a few vitamins that can cause some problems if taken in too high a dose. Vitamin B6 is known to produce some neurological symptoms in doses of 100mg or more a day. The need for fat-soluble Vitamin A varies, and a higher-protein diet can increase the need for Vitamin A. Doses of Vitamin A higher than 100,000 IU a day for more than a month should be monitored by a knowledgeable practitioner. Likewise, Vitamin D3 levels should be monitored with blood tests to ensure that you are staying in the recommended range. We need a *balance* of Vitamins A, D, and K, as they work synergistically.

TAKING VITAMINS AND OTHER SUPPLEMENTS:

Avoid those with chemical fillers.

Some vitamin companies) ensure high standards, but not all do. (See Appendix for details)

Remember, vitamins should be taken *with a meal.* When the process of digestion is already in action, the vitamins are more likely to be adequately broken down and absorbed.

"Are there situations that hold special needs for vitamins?" Gastric-bypass surgery and colon surgery drastically affect digestion and the ability to absorb nutrients from food. Stomach stapling, or gastric-bypass surgery, means that most of your stomach is gone. The food's ability to be broken down by stomach acid before entering the small intestine is very limited. If part of the small intestine has also been disconnected, the available absorption space is reduced. Certain vitamins, such as B12, depend on binding with intrinsic factors in the stomach and are only absorbed in the terminal part of the ileum—which is no longer present after gastric-bypass surgery. If part of the colon has been removed, then fewer nutrients are absorbed before the stool passes out of the body.

A number of pharmaceutical drugs also interfere with vitamin uptake and can create deficiencies. It is important to research any drugs that you are taking and supplement them appropriately to prevent any potential vitamin loss.

In these cases, closer monitoring of vitamin levels is warranted. Most laboratories measure the amount of vitamins by looking in the liquid (serum) part of the blood. However, this only measures the amount dissolved in the blood. What we really want to know is how well the vitamins and minerals are *getting into the cells*.

I use special tests designed by Spectracell Laboratories that evaluate the level of vitamins and minerals that the white blood cells have actually absorbed. Spectracell takes the white blood cells and plates them onto nutrient material, each of which is missing one vitamin or mineral. If the white blood cells have not absorbed enough zinc, for example, then the cells growing in the zinc-deficient media will not grow as well as those in the control media, which has all the nutrients. The measure of reduced growth is reported as a level of deficiency of that nutrient. This kind of test is very helpful in developing an appropriate vitamin supplementation plan, and also in following up to see if the plan is effective.

"What Should I Know about Herbal Products?"

I recommend buying herbs from reputable companies. With herbs that have been ground up and put into *capsules*, the age of the product is important: such herbs will lose their medicinal vitality more quickly. Herbs that have been made into alcohol-based *tinctures*, in contrast, remain stable much longer. Some herbs can also be effectively used fresh or dried, in teas or food. Herbs work in quantity, so the amount makes a difference. You want to use enough of them and often enough to get the desired effect. But note that it also is possible to use too much of an herb.

When I was a medical resident, a patient came to our clinic who had taken a *pound* of dried yohimbe (an herb touted to help libido). He had boiled it down and then drunk the entire amount. The man had selected the herb for its aphrodisiac effect; however, the amount he had consumed had the effect of greatly over-stimulating his entire nervous system. His blood pressure was 200 something over 100 something; his heart rate was elevated; he was sweating; and he hadn't been able to sleep for several days. He felt like he was jumping out of his skin. Sexual pleasure was *not* on his mind by the time we saw him.

It is a good idea to work with an experienced herbalist, someone familiar with and trained in herbal medicine. There are also many wonderful books available that can help you learn about the uses of specific herbs. I recommend using herbs that are organically grown or wildcrafted. "Wildcrafted" means that the plants are not cultivated but are picked growing in the wild. Certain wildcrafting rules need to be followed, such as: picking less that 10 percent of the total number of plants in the area; picking neither the smallest nor the largest specimens, but instead choosing those in the middle range; picking in the appropriate season and time of day for that plant; and not picking plants that grow close to major highways or other sources of pollution.

HERBS

Use enough and often enough (but not too much) to get the desired effect.

Tinctures retain their vitality longer than ground herbs.

Fresh or dried herbs work well in teas and food.

Consider working with an experienced herbalist, or read informative books.

Healthy Breakfast, Lunch, and Dinner Suggestions

"What is a *good* breakfast?" A good breakfast should have some protein, some fat, and some fiber. Protein and fat break down into blood sugar much more slowly compared to carbohydrates. A good breakfast looks a lot like what Grandpa and Grandma ate back on the farm: whole eggs (not egg whites only), preferably cooked in butter; good bacon, scrapple, or sausage from a pastured pig (preferably without the nitrates, sugar, and other additives); and perhaps a slice of genuine sourdough toast with butter.

Bread, if you choose to eat it, should be dense, one that must be chewed—the kind of bread you could sit on and it would hold its

> **A GOOD BREAKFAST:**
>
> Should include some protein, some fat, and some fiber.
>
> ✦
>
> Grains like oats should be soaked overnight.

shape—not something labeled "whole-grain" but with the texture of Wonder Bread.

Some people like hot oatmeal for breakfast. Oatmeal can be fine if it is not instant and doesn't have added sugar or artificial flavors. Oats need to be soaked overnight before cooking, otherwise they can be quite toxic. Other grains can also be soaked overnight, and then cooked for breakfast. You can add some peanut butter or almond butter and some butter or coconut oil, or heavy cream instead of milk. That will increase the protein and fat content in the meal. Sweeten with fruit, maple syrup, or honey, if desired. That should hold you until lunchtime.

"**What do you suggest for lunch?**" A good lunch consists of protein, fat, and veggies. Some people like sandwiches for lunch, and find themselves at a loss if they are cutting back on bread. Good alternatives might be tuna (or chicken, or mackerel or canned salmon) mixed with a good amount of whole-fat mayonnaise, together with some cooked veggies (leftovers?), or a nice salad with a full-fat dressing. If I'm in a hurry, I might choose an apple, sliced thinly, with heaping amounts of peanut or almond butter (at least 2 or 3 tablespoonfuls). Or open a can of sardines, preferably containing the skin and bones, so you get the benefit of the added calcium and fat. Leftover homemade soup, cheeses, and pâté are also great lunch items.

Remember—fat is not the enemy! We *need* fat in our food to support our brain function and steady our metabolism. And fat is especially important for young, growing children. I have a friend who is a full-fat cook. She says it's too confusing for people to have this important nutrient bear the same name as the common word for obesity. She thinks fat needs a new name, like "God's Nectar."

When the weather is cold, I like to make up a big stew of chicken (whole, with skin and bones) with a bone-broth base, adding veggies such as celery, carrots, parsnips, turnips, garlic, onion, and maybe some ginger.

I make a big pot for dinner and heat some up for lunch the next day. For variety, I make a stew based on beef, pork, or lamb instead of chicken. When I heat it up, I add chopped collards, mustard, kale, or Swiss chard to get my greens in. If I don't have any greens, sometimes I'll just add some organic salad mix. In cold weather, I find the cooked greens much more palatable than cold salad.

A GOOD LUNCH SHOULD INCLUDE:

Protein (chicken, pâté; tuna, mackerel, salmon, sardines with skin and bones; nut butters; cheese; etc.)

✦

Fat (whole-fat mayonnaise, full-fat dressing, etc.) Remember—Fat is not the enemy!

✦

Veggies (soup, leftovers, etc.)

"**And what should I eat for dinner?**" **Preventing blood-sugar drop:** Many of the patients I see work long hours and spend an additional couple of hours on their commute. They don't get home until late, six or more hours after they ate lunch. Since keeping a steady blood sugar means that you need to eat protein and fat about every four hours, I suggest that these people have a hearty snack—not a protein bar (which often are sweet), but hard-boiled eggs with some mayo, apples with nut butter, or "Energy Balls" about four hours after lunch. (See the Appendix at the end of the book for the Energy Balls recipe.) This prevents their blood sugar from bottoming out by the time they get home, so they are less likely to reach for the high-carb snack foods to tide them over. If they happen to stop for gas on the way home and get tempted, I tell them to get fried pork rinds and some cashews, sunflower seeds, or peanuts rather than chips or popcorn. Remember, the key is eating protein and fat every four hours to keep your blood sugar and energy steady.

Cooking ahead: Some of my patients have found that it helps to cook a bunch of dinners ahead of time on Saturday or Sunday. Then throughout the week they can just heat up what they already have cooked—and *voila,* dinner is ready! The crockpot can be a real ally. Try sticking a whole or cut chicken (or brisket, seafood, or pork-shoulder roast) in, along with salt and pepper, some veggies, onion, and garlic. Then turn the crockpot on low before you leave home in the morning. Dinner will be done and ready to eat by the time you return. The Instapot has shortened cooking time, and made stews, soups, and roasts even easier to make from scratch.

Many root veggies are just as tasty made ahead and then heated up for dinner. The same is true for greens such as kale, collards, and chard, sautéed in butter, coconut oil, or bacon fat. These veggies store well in the refrigerator. They add a lovely variety of colors, tastes, and textures, as well as providing a good source of insoluble fiber.

We need that insoluble fiber to add bulk to our stool and help us stay regular.

COOK AHEAD:

Cook once / eat more than one time.

→

Crockpot meals + veggies (sautéed or roasted) keep you well fed, healthy, and regular.

Gluten

We've been hearing a lot about gluten. Many people are choosing to go gluten-free, these days. The supermarkets are suddenly full of gluten-free items. It's not hard to find gluten-free bread, muffins, crackers, cereals—even pop tarts!—in every grocery store today.

EAT HEALTHY, HEARTY SNACKS:

to stabilize blood sugar = protein + fat every 4 hours!

Gluten is a general name for the proteins found in wheat (durum, emmer, spelt, farina, farro, kamut, khorasan, and einkorn), rye, barley, and triticale. Gluten helps baked foods to maintain their shape, and makes dough more elastic and stretchy.

A note of caution: If your goal is to become healthier and/or lose weight, just substituting gluten-free products for the gluten-containing processed foods you are now eating *will not help*. The clever food industry has climbed on the gluten-free wagon and is having a field day. Many of the gluten-free products are made largely with rice starch, potato starch, cornstarch, or tapioca starch. These are foods that will raise your blood sugar just as quickly and as high, or possibly higher, than wheat! Don't go down that path! Avoid the gluten-*free* pasta, cereal and bread, as well as the gluten-*containing* pasta and bread. They are all high-glycemic foods.

"Am I gluten-intolerant?" You may not be aware of whether gluten affects you or not. One way to find out is to choose to eliminate *all high-gluten foods* from your diet for a month. Grains high in gluten include: wheat (and all varieties, such as durum, emmer, spelt, farina, farro, kamut, khorasan wheat, and einkorn), rye, and barley. It takes a month at least to fully remove the impact of gluten from your body. A few days are not enough. The best solution is to set a start date and just quit eating *any* gluten.

Some of my patients notice that when they stop eating wheat, they find themselves craving it. This is because some of the constituents in the *new* wheat (i.e., not the wheat grown a generation and more ago) act almost like opiates with some people. And if you cheat and have a little, you may find yourself craving more. Other people find that they feel really sick if they cheat.

However, some of my patients who changed to gluten-free foods were surprised to notice that their muscle or joint pains stopped, their bowels and stomach worked better, their skin problems disappeared, and their minds became clearer. The only way to know how wheat affects you is to eliminate it and see the effects. You can still have the burger, but set aside the bun. Roll your sandwiches in a lettuce leaf, instead. Have corn chips (organic) instead of wheat crackers, and a non-wheat cereal instead of Wheaties. If you eat a lot of processed foods, you will need to become a label-reader. I carry reading glasses when I shop so that I can decipher all that fine print in the Ingredients list on the packaging. Wheat comes in canned soups, sauces, salad dressings, and a myriad of prepared products that you may find yourself surprised to discover.

"Do I have a gluten allergy?" Another way to find out if gluten is a problem for you is to get some testing for gluten antibodies and gliadin (another protein found in wheat) antibodies. Make sure that the test includes the antibodies IgA and IgG as well as IgE. The IgG and IgA antibodies are involved in delayed sensitivity reactions. Delayed sensitivity reactions can occur hours to days after exposure to gluten, so they are much more difficult to detect by simple observation.

"Do I have celiac disease if gluten bothers me?" Many people are confused between *gluten sensitivity* and *Celiac disease*. Celiac disease is a medical term diagnosed by the presence of anti-tissue transglutaminase antibodies (anti tTG), and atrophy of the villi (hairlike projections) in the small intestine. In order to know if the small intestines have atrophied, a sample has to be taken during an endoscopy. Also, if you have already been avoiding wheat or high-gluten foods for a while, your intestines may have recovered and will no longer appear atrophied.

I have seen a number of people who were well aware of digestive problems due to wheat, yet they tested negative for celiac disease after undergoing endoscopies and blood tests. The changes in the wheat grown today is causing problems in people who do not have Celiac disease.

Unfortunately, most conventional allergists and other physicians test for food allergies only by looking at IgE antibodies to foods. The IgE antibody is only involved in *immediate* allergic reactions. As a result, many people who have gone to allergists and had testing have been told, "You don't have any food allergies. It's all in your mind." They may very well have specific delayed sensitivity reactions to certain foods, including gluten, but the tests that were done were not adequate.

Most people are already aware of their immediate allergic reactions and don't need IgE antibody testing. They are already avoiding those things that trigger early reactions.

What allergists are doing with IgE testing is like looking under the streetlight for lost keys, when it was down in the dark alley that the keys were lost. They are looking in the wrong place. You need to find a doctor who knows how to do the appropriate food-allergy testing. Some food-allergy tests can also be found online. The Appendix contains a list of some laboratories that conduct food allergy tests.

"What *is* the problem with wheat?" I'm going to say again what I said in Chapter Two on digestion, because it's important enough to bear repeating: *today's wheat is different from the wheat that Grandma and Grandpa ate a generation or two ago.*

Growing up in Kansas, I saw beautiful wheat fields with long, tall, pale-gold stalks and large seed-heads. If a big storm came just before harvest time, those heavy heads of wheat would fill with water and become sodden, and the whole wheat field would be bent over because the stalks weren't able to bear the water's weight. This meant that a farmer could lose his whole harvest in a single night.

This has changed. In the 1960s and '70s, scientists began to use hybridization methods to develop a new kind of wheat: much shorter (only about 18 to 22 inches tall), with a dark-brownish color, and stronger stalks that can withstand rainstorms and drought and give a higher yield. Gone are the waving fields of pale gold wheat that I remember from childhood. This new wheat will not be destroyed by a late-season storm, so it's less of a risk for the farmers. It has been designed specifically to have more of the qualities desired for both growing and baking purposes. To satisfy the bakers' requests, the new wheat has more gluten than ever before.

This newly engineered wheat also contains hundreds of unique compounds never before encountered by humans, and our bodies are responding differently to it. Even *pigs* are reported to have problems with the new wheat. And this wheat is grown worldwide; only small pockets of older strains are still grown—in southern France, parts of Italy, and the Middle East. (For more details about the changes in wheat and the effects on humans, see the Appendix for what Dr. William Davis has written in his book, *Wheatbelly*.)

My own journey without wheat began when I noticed that after eating pasta, I experienced mental dullness and physical sluggishness. Gradually, I chose to eat less and less pasta. When I stopped entirely, I discovered that I felt full and satisfied without the heavy feeling in my belly that pasta seemed to create. When I noticed that same heavy feeling after eating pizza, I began to eat less pizza. This evolved into letting go of bread, and finding other ways of eating without toast, crackers. and sandwiches.

About a year or two ago I stopped eating all grains and beans and starchy vegetables to see how I felt. That's when I noticed the biggest change: not only was my mind clearer and my energy more sustained, but my whole body felt somehow lighter, more *lithe*, and I noticed that my clothes became looser. Today, I eat low-gluten grains and beans occasionally and in moderation, and continue to feel good.

Special Concerns: Diabetes

Diabetes has become a raging epidemic in the U.S. and much of the Western world. Instead of targeting the widespread promotion of fast convenience foods and sweet drinks in creating this epidemic, doctors and public health officials seem to blame the victim. It's time for public health officials and doctors to speak out about the lack of social responsibility that the food industry displays in promoting these non-nutritious, highly profitable, and health-killing products. The failure to raise public awareness about the health dangers these "foods" present speaks to a lack of social responsibility on the part of the medical profession, as well.

Let's talk about blood sugar: We are all unique individuals with biochemical individuality, each with our own unique set of genetic predispositions. If you have a number of relatives who *developed* diabetes—not the kind that you are born with, but Type 2 diabetes, which develops later in life—you may have inherited a tendency to metabolize blood sugar differently from the majority of people. In some families, no one went to the doctor until they were at death's door, so no one knew if they had diabetes or not.

Another clue that you may have inherited this different blood-sugar metabolism is if there is a strong tendency towards alcoholism in your family. Many alcoholics have an underlying blood-sugar metabolism "wobble," which allows them to drink large quantities of alcohol (a simple carbohydrate) without experiencing its sedative effects. They can sustain their alcoholic high for hours. Those of us without this blood-sugar "wobble" find that after two or three drinks, we are so sedated that we just want to go to sleep. And usually we do just that.

Medically speaking, diabetes is diagnosed when blood-sugar levels are consistently elevated. However, blood-sugar metabolism problems can be detected and corrected *years earlier* by checking the fasting and postprandial (after-eating) blood levels of insulin.

"How does insulin work?" Insulin is produced in the pancreas. It acts like a doorman, opening the cell's door to allow the glucose in the blood to enter the cell where it is needed and be used for fuel. People who are genetically predisposed to develop diabetes have a pancreas that is capable of becoming an *over*producer of insulin. Their pancreas is hyper-reactive to blood-sugar levels; and over time, if they persist in eating a high-carbohydrate diet, the pancreas puts out more and more insulin in response to the surges of blood sugar.

This results in several significant consequences.

One is that, as the level of insulin rises over the years, the cells develop resistance to the insulin. Because of this resistance, it takes more and more insulin to open the cell's door and move the blood sugar into the cells. (The doorman needs more and more muscle to open the cell's door.) This continues until one day, the cells simply won't let the blood sugar in at all. The blood sugar then remains in the blood and gets higher and higher over time. This is the point at which the medical profession diagnoses "diabetes."

I have never understood why doctors are not taught to monitor the fasting *insulin*. An elevated fasting insulin level is a sure predictor that the person will develop diabetes if they do not change their eating patterns and choice of foods. What doctors usually test is the fasting *glucose*, or the Hemoglobin A1C (HgA1C). The HgA1C reflects the average blood-sugar level over the previous six weeks. It is a more accurate picture of blood-sugar levels than a random fasting blood-glucose level alone.

"What does diabetes do to the body?" The damage begins when the amount of sugar in the blood starts to rise above normal. Elevated levels of blood sugar act like a corrosive agent on the blood-vessel walls. This is especially damaging for the tiniest blood vessels, called capillaries, which are only a single-cell thick. Their walls were meant to act like semi-permeable membranes, allowing nutrients to pass through their walls into the cells and allowing waste material to pass from the cell back into the blood, where it is transported to be removed from the body. High levels of blood sugar effectively sandblast the walls of the capillaries, and the membranes become thickened and less permeable. This means that the cells that surround them can neither get the nutrients they need nor release the toxins and accumulated wastes that need to be removed.

Diabetes is called "The Silent Killer" because the usual warning signs of body injury (e.g., pain or bleeding) do not occur. Over time, as the capillary walls thicken, the cells they serve become less functional, and eventually they die. The areas that suffer first are the ones most dependent on those tiny capillaries: the retina of the eye; the fingers and toes; and the kidneys. The kidneys are basically massive amounts of capillaries that serve as the body's major filtration system. So, over time, the retina doesn't work very well and vision is impaired. I know one man whose blood sugars had been high probably since his teens, but he had not sought medical care until he became legally blind in his forties. He had high blood sugar for many years and never knew it.

When the capillaries in the fingers and toes don't function well, people develop neuropathy, which means that the nerve cells stop functioning properly. A diabetic can literally walk around with a thumbtack stuck on the bottom of his foot and not feel the pain, because the nerve cells in his foot aren't working. Cuts don't heal well, and may not even be noticed unless the feet are examined very carefully on a regular basis. The damaged capillaries have undermined the body's pain-signaling system, due to the elevated blood sugar. Over time, the kidneys stop being able to function as the blood's filtration system. Ultimately, the diabetic may require dialysis in order to keep from being self-poisoned. And as anyone who has had to go on dialysis can tell you, it means spending many hours several times a week, immobile and hooked up to a machine to filter your blood. Not a happy picture.

"How can I tell if I have a blood-sugar problem?" For patients who already have been told that their blood sugar is a bit high, this is a clue that they have a problem with blood-sugar metabolism. Women who were diagnosed with gestational diabetes during pregnancy were given a heads-up that they have an underlying blood-sugar metabolism wobble. If you have a family history of diabetes or alcoholism, that is another clue that you might have a problem.

Sometimes, hypoglycemia can be a clue. People who have hypoglycemia know that they have to eat at regular intervals in order to maintain equilibrium. If they go too long without eating, they become very irritable, tired, shaky, and/or find it difficult to concentrate. A good cure for hypoglycemia is to avoid sweets and to eat a good amount of fat, especially saturated animal fat, every four hours.

The best way to detect a blood-sugar problem early is to check your fasting insulin with a blood test. If it is more than 11, you are on the road to developing diabetes unless you change what you are eating.

"How do I check my insulin level?" Get a blood test for insulin after you have fasted for at least six hours. Once the fasting insulin has been checked and found to be high, it's time to look at what you eat. My patients and I go over each entry in their food log and look for the simple carbohydrates—in plain language, the starchy stuff: the bread, pop tarts, muffins, breakfast cereals, crackers, chips, pretzels, cookies, and candy. These foods are made from grains that have been processed (ground into a fine powder), and often there are added sugars, as well. And don't forget the breading on deep-fried foods!

"Why does the Standard American Diet promote diabetes?" The typical SAD breakfast (if *any* breakfast is eaten at all) is usually some cereal with low-fat milk and maybe some juice, or a toaster waffle or pop tart. Sometimes it's a protein bar (aka, a candy bar with added soy), or a piece of toast or a donut grabbed as you rush out the door. All of these products contain mostly refined carbohydrates.

Almost all boxed cereals are refined carbohydrates. Whether it calls itself "whole-grain" or not, it is made by crushing grains into a fine powder and adding liquid to create a pulp, which is then extruded into various shapes. Extrusion warps the proteins in the grains. These extruded cereals also create problems in the gut flora.

Grain that has been ground into a powder has been turned into a simple carbohydrate that breaks down very quickly into blood sugar in the body. The quick breakdown will cause a big surge in blood sugar within an hour after eating. This rapid surge of blood sugar stimulates insulin levels to rise. Insulin rushes out to act like a doorman, opening the cell's door to allow blood sugar (technically known as *glucose*) to enter the cell. The cell uses the glucose as its fuel to make ATP, the form of energy that drives the cell's other biochemical reactions.

When blood levels of insulin surge after a high-carbohydrate meal such as cereal, pancakes, juice, waffles, or sweetened non-fat yogurt, there are also other consequences. The insulin surge helps the blood sugar move rapidly into the cells. That results in an equally rapid drop of sugar levels in the blood. The bigger the insulin surge, the quicker the drop in blood sugar. This process takes roughly two hours. The result is that two hours after a high-carbohydrate meal, the brain is signaling, "Quick—blood sugar is getting low, we need to eat something RIGHT NOW!" Many people have told me that they feel hungry again two hours after a high-carbohydrate meal.

Insulin also sends messages to the liver as to the status of the body's wellbeing. An insulin level that fluctuates widely between lows and highs sends the message, "We cannot rely on a steady intake of food—conditions are rapidly fluctuating—so prepare for survival." In response, the liver begins to store every spare calorie. Calories are stored as cholesterol and glycogen. The result is that the liver produces excess cholesterol (a quickly produced storage form of blood sugar) in the blood and increased amounts of glycogen, which are stored as the fat on our hips, midsections, buttocks, and thighs as well as in the liver itself.

"Why do I have fatty liver?" Fatty liver is another result of maintaining a higher blood-sugar level over time. Fatty liver is a condition in which the liver is storing the excess calories as fat within its own tissue. What is more, a widely fluctuating insulin level, with its message of an unstable and unreliable food source, also causes our metabolism or the burning of calories to be reduced in an effort to conserve whatever fuel we have on board. When the thermostat is turned down, we burn calories more slowly. No wonder people on high-carbohydrate diets have so much trouble losing weight!

Refined carbohydrates (e.g., cereal, crackers, bread, tortillas, or rice cakes) break down into blood sugar quickly, and within two hours the blood sugar has moved into the cells. That is why people who have the SAD breakfast find that they are hungry about two hours after they have eaten. Their brain is signaling them that they have reached a critically low blood sugar, and they must act fast. If they are at the office, they might grab a quick snack, or stop and get a snack at a fast-food place, or grab that candy bar in the car. The intake of another simple carbohydrate will quickly replenish the body's blood-sugar supply. But as we know, it also starts another turn on the same cycle of rapidly alternating high and low blood-sugar and insulin levels.

"How can I avoid diabetes?" If you have a hyperactive pancreas and your food intake is high in "simple carbohydrates" (foods that break down into blood sugar very quickly), you are triggering these high-insulin releases on a regular basis. Even if you have a normal-functioning pancreas but are eating mostly refined carbohydrates, you can develop abnormally high levels of insulin. If this pattern continues over time, you are hastening the development of insulin resistance and, eventually, diabetes. Often, elevated fasting-insulin levels can be detected *years* before frank diabetes develops.

As I said before, I have never understood why most physicians never check the fasting insulin but only the fasting blood glucose. The ideal fasting insulin should be 11 or less. I have seen patients with fasting-insulin levels in the 20s and 30s. These people are well on their way to developing diabetes, due to insulin-resistance. Unless they make some big changes in their food choices now, eventually they will be told that they have developed diabetes. At that point, the choices for treatment become more limited, and they may need to resort to drugs to maintain normal blood-sugar levels. By the time they are diagnosed with diabetes, many people have already developed irreversible damage in their capillaries. The "Silent Killer" has already begun its work.

"But isn't a whole-grain cereal good for me?" That breakfast cereal labeled "'whole-grain" may indeed have started out as a whole-grain or grains. However, those grains were then ground into a powder, to which various binders, preservatives (such as BHT), sweeteners (such as high-fructose corn syrup, dextrose, glucose, or artificial sweeteners like aspartame or sorbitol), and artificial flavors and colors were added.

The same is true for pasta and breads labeled "whole grain." If they consist of finely ground flour, they have become simple carbohydrates. They no longer have the nutritional value of whole grains in them anymore.

Our *bodies* can't read the label that says "whole-grain." What they experience is a processed starch that breaks down into blood sugar very quickly. The rapid rise in blood sugar then stimulates a big surge in insulin. Obviously, those cereals that also have added sugars will raise the blood sugar even more. You can find the list of added sugars by reading the *Ingredients list* on the package, not the "Nutrition Facts."

What, then, should you do?

If you *prepare* the whole grain—whether brown rice, whole-wheat berries, millet, etc.—by first soaking it overnight, draining that water off, and then cooking it, you will get the benefits of the whole grain. However, to make a *complete* breakfast, you want to add some fat—butter, coconut oil, or sour cream—and some protein, such as nut butters, or eat it with sausage or bacon.

> *The key to good nutrition is to pay attention to*
> *your body and notice what nourishes it.*
> *Find your nourishing rhythm, and dance.*

CHAPTER FOUR

EXERCISE OR VITALIZE?

The Rhythm of Work and Play

"It does not matter how slowly you go, so long as you do not stop."
—CONFUCIUS

There's something about the word *exercise* that I don't like. It holds the energy of a drill sergeant. There's a hidden reproach in it. I've heard so many people say, "I *should* exercise" or "I don't exercise *enough*." It's rare that I meet a person who feels good about exercise and their relationship to it.

So when I sit together with my patients, I don't even ask them about exercise. Instead I say, "Tell me what kind of *activity* you do in your day."

Our bodies are constantly in motion. We are not statues. *Movement enlivens and vitalizes the body.* Finding our own unique rhythm through our movements each day is key to feeling vital and alive. Our bodies were intended to *move*, to be *active*, to feel *alive*. How we go about fully realizing our enlivened potential is as individual as our fingerprints.

Find what grounds you—and gives you a sense of play.

People today are as confused about exercise as they are about food. We are barraged by promotions for weight training, bodybuilding, kickboxing, boot camps, marathons, Jazzercise, Zumba, Pilates, and more. The result is an environment of confusion, frustration, and shame.

We can start to unravel the confusion a bit by sorting out the distinctions among three very different concepts: movement, activity, and exercise.

Movement is a Core Rhythm of life. Without movement, there *is* no life. Movement is aliveness. It is internal and external, physical, mental, emotional, and spiritual. It is the business of living. From the moment we are born until we take our last breath, we move.

Activity is something we do by choice. It could be window shopping or window washing. It could be walking the dog or riding a bike. Activity is something we choose to do and often enjoy.

Exercise is intentional activity that is done with specific goals regarding physical endurance, and improvement and maintenance of strength, mobility, and stability. The word "exercise" carries a lot of baggage with it. We are bombarded with directives about what kind of exercise we *should* be doing. Our culture has an obsession with extremes. Exercise has become conflated with the idea of attaining a "perfect" body. TV programs like "Extreme Makeover Weight Loss Edition" and "The Biggest Loser" feed the fantasy.

Choosing to exercise in the hopes of attaining the "perfect" body is a quest that is bound to end in defeat. Many of us already know this, yet we continue to buy into the fantasy. If we don't quit and yet we haven't achieved our fantasied perfection, we feel cheated. If we quit, then we feel shame. There are no happy endings to this story.

Let's look at it from a *holistic* approach.

The first thing we need to do is rethink or reshape our attitude towards physical activity. I'm not talking about an Extreme Makeover. I'm suggesting that we take a deep breath and release all the *shoulds* we have accumulated regarding exercise. Let go of the "I *should* exercise more" and the 'I *should* have a regular exercise program I follow," etc. Let go of *all* the *shoulds*. Deep inhale. Deep exhale. Let it go.

Good. Now, let's begin.

When Did Human Beings Stop Moving?

> "Dancers are so much happier than dieters and exercisers.... Perfection is 'lean' and 'taut' and 'hard'—like a boy athlete of twenty, a girl gymnast of twelve.... 'Perfect'? What's perfect? There are a whole lot of ways to be perfect, and not one of them is attained through punishment."
>
> —Ursula K. Le Guin

Today, few of us still need to chop wood and carry water, or even hang out the wash on a clothesline. It is only in recent history—the last few generations—that we humans began to spend most of our waking hours virtually stationary. We *sit* and commute to work, where we *sit* at a desk; we *sit* on the way home, and then we *sit* in front of the TV or computer until we go to bed. Some say sitting has become the new smoking.

Physical activity—moving—is something that our bodies were built to do. Remember when you were a kid? Did your mother or father *make* you play? Or was it something you just did because it was fun, it felt good, and you wanted to do it? Children are naturally physically active, each according to their own nature. Trying to keep a child from playing is like trying to stop a river from flowing.

We don't lose that innate need for joyful play as we get older, even though we may learn to sit still and be quiet when it's expected. We've been conditioned since kindergarten to sit still, so we're working to undo many years of conditioning, here.

In my high school, only the "dumb kids" got to move—go to shop class, learn automechanics, and have real jobs. The "smart kids" didn't have to move their bodies. So we didn't, unless we happened to be one of the few on a sports team. The rest of us just pretty much stopped moving.

The key to *vitalizing* is to find the activities that bring you *joy* as well as keep you moving. And only *you* are the best judge of what those activities are, no one else. The specific activities that you choose are not as important as the regular *doing* of it—daily, if possible. Let joyous movement become another daily rhythm in your life, like eating and sleeping.

When I ask my patients, "What kind of physical activity do you get on a daily basis?" it's rare that I hear a contented response. I've lost count of how many times I hear, "I know I *should* exercise more," or "I *used* to run," or "I'm *planning* on joining a gym as soon as I have time." Just by listening, I can sense the self-condemnation, shame, or guilt they are carrying. Sometimes, there is also a note of wistfulness as they acknowledge that they find themselves not doing what they would like to be doing.

WHAT DO YOU *LIKE* TO DO?

"I know I should exercise," one patient told me, sighing. "I even have a gym in my basement. But it's so boring!"

"I understand," I commiserated with her. "I have a hard time with repetitive-motion machines myself. Are there any physical activities that you enjoy doing? "

"I would love to play *ping pong* with my husband!" she exclaimed suddenly. "And we already have a ping pong table in our house!" Her whole face lit up at the thought.

Another patient responded, "Oh, I love *dancing!*" Suddenly she began thinking of ways to put more dancing in her life, and the thought that she could increase her physical activity by dancing put a smile on her face.

The point is to find your *own* rhythm of movement: find what activity brings *you* joy. Think back to when you were a child. What did you enjoy doing?

- Did you like the feeling of being outside?

- Or was it nice to be indoors, lying on the floor and moving?

- Did you like being in the water?

- Playing with a ball?

- Roller skating?

- Dancing to music?

- Dancing in the rain?

- Or _____?

Some people like bird watching—but spotting the birds is the bonus. For them, it's also about walking in the woods or on a beach. Some enjoy fishing. Maybe you'll catch a fish; but maybe you'll walk down the bank (while the rod sits there, poised), take a little stroll, and explore.

You don't have to play golf to spend an afternoon outside. But you *could* play golf. Or croquet. Some people like rebounder balls—giant balls you can sit on and bounce on while you play video games or catch up on Facebook. Sitting on a ball keeps your body much more engaged than if you were just sitting on a chair. You have to keep moving to stay on the ball. You can even move in rhythm to music, if you like. Your body is actively engaged in maintaining your position, which needs constant tweaking. I know a writer who writes while walking on her treadmill.

My point is: *find what movement or activity grounds you—and gives you a sense of play.*

Moving our bodies to maintain body strength and tone has become something we must consciously plan and program into our already overly busy schedules. But it also can be more improvisational. For instance, you can simply park farther from work in order to walk more, take the stairs, walk during your lunch hour, stand at your desk, or sit on a balance ball. All these changes are helpful.

GETTING HAPPILY STARTED

How much activity do you need? For most people, moving their body for a half hour each day is a good goal. I use the term "moving" rather than "exercise" because there are many different ways you can choose to move your body. It could look like walking, or dancing, or yoga, or raking leaves, or something else that you enjoy doing. The point is to be moving *and* enjoying yourself.

Many of you have already noticed what a great stress-reliever physical activity can be. Getting outdoors, moving, and shifting your focus can lift mountains of tension off your shoulders. Allow yourself a break, stretch the collagen, and change your pace. Even ten minutes of movement can breathe new life into your day. Some studies have shown that daily walking works faster, and sometimes better, than antidepressants like Prozac.

Many companies have discovered that physical activity increases their employees' productivity. These enlightened companies provide onsite gym equipment, yoga, and other exercise classes, and some even have massage therapists available.

When I worked in a busy primary-care office with patients scheduled every fifteen minutes, I made an amazing discovery. Since my schedule included an hour break for lunch every day, I joined a nearby gym with a pool. The days I left the office, swam for twenty minutes, and returned in time to eat my lunch and be ready for my next patient, I found that I had more energy for the rest of the day. Sometimes I chose to stay at the office during lunch because the amount of catch-up work seemed overwhelming. Yet I noticed that the same amount of work got done whether I took a break and exercised or not. And the bonus was that when I exercised I felt more relaxed, more alert, and better able to focus.

My daughter Molly, an experienced personal trainer, says it's important to set goals before you start to help you stay focused and give you a real sense of accomplishment. She emphasizes that the goals should be specific, like "Lose X pounds" or "Touch my toes" rather than "Lose weight" or "Be more flexible." Goals should also be realistic. If you've been sedentary for the past few years, setting a goal of running a marathon in two months or joining a boot-camp class is not realistic.

Stretching, Warm-Ups, and Cool-Downs

Before you start, don't forget to stretch and warm up! This is very important, especially if you haven't been very active for a while. Stretching, along with cool-downs and warm-ups, helps to prevent lactic-acid buildup in the muscles. Lactic-acid buildup in muscles makes them ache and feel sore after a workout. If you get too sore the first time you are active, you may avoid moving the next day because of discomfort—the equivalent of shooting yourself in the foot.

Warms-ups activate the muscles and let the body know that it is time to do work. A good warm-up activity mimics the exercise you intend to do: air squats before applying weight, or tossing a medicine ball before an upper-body workout, enable the blood to begin flowing toward the muscles that will be working, bringing with it needed oxygen. Cool-downs are equally important to return the body to its resting state, distribute lactic acid out of the muscles, and stretch out tight tissues to increase flexibility. Cool-downs are a great opportunity to address any typical issues (such as a bum shoulder) with correctional stretching and working out tissue adhesions and knots.

Active, or *dynamic,* stretching is good to warm up; and *static* stretching after working out will improve overall flexibility and alignment. Active stretching involves movements such as rolling your shoulders or doing knee bends. Static stretching means holding a stretch for at least 30 seconds. You will see increased flexibility in as little as four weeks of doing 30-second holds.

If you are just beginning to exercise, do it in moderation. This means that if you have not been walking, start with five or ten minutes a day and slowly build up to thirty minutes. Remember the story of the tortoise and the hare? Slow and steady is the name of the game. Start small and basic before moving on to more complicated moves.

*Slow and steady is the name of the game. Start
small and basic before moving on to more
complicated moves.*

"How Do I Avoid Injuries?"

Before beginning any strenuous exercise or workout program, get a physical exam. Make sure that your body is *ready* to be more active. It may also benefit you to consult a personal trainer or another expert to lead you through exercises and ensure that you are performing them correctly. Performing exercise with bad form can lead to problematic injuries.

Correct and Strengthen the Weak Areas

Nothing is more discouraging than to start an exercise program and then have to stop because of an injury. The best predictor of future injury is past injury. If you have sprained an ankle or had a knee or shoulder injury, that part of your body is inherently weaker and more likely to get re-injured.

The weakened area needs *correction* first, and then *strengthening*. Even if you haven't suffered a previous injury, it is extremely important to make sure that any underlying structural problems are corrected before beginning any vigorous activity. Someone whose shoulder, spine, hips, knees, or ankles are out of alignment or structurally disorganized has a set-up just waiting for injuries to happen. This is especially true if you start doing repetitive-motion exercises.

People with a weak knee, a bad ankle, or back problems may have re-injured these areas in the past when suddenly initiating a strenuous exercise program. I have found that attending to these vulnerable conditions before initiating any strenuous activity program is important to avoid more injury.

Many of these conditions exist because of underlying structural disorganization. There are many trained body workers who can help to re-organize and re-align the body's structure. These include physical therapists, trainers who are CES (Corrective Exercise Specialists), Rolfers, myofascial release therapists, Feldenkreis, Alexander technique, Trager work, chiropractors, cranial osteopaths, cranio-sacral therapists, and others.

A word of caution: Do not attempt to start a new *strenuous* program of activity *until you are sure you are well aligne*d. Correcting any structural problems and resolving any outstanding injuries is key to maintain health-building physical activity.

Don't Be a "Weekend Warrior"

The weekend-warrior approach—with strenuous exercise on the weekend, and nothing in between—can be another recipe for disaster. You are more likely to sustain an injury from intermittent hard exercise than from more gentle daily movement. There is no dishonor in approaching the basics first. No one started out as an amazing weight lifter, runner, or athlete; and the great athletes know the importance of going back to basic movements from time to time. Complexity is not always an indication of a better exercise.

Some people get inspired to start exercising and make the mistake of going from couch-potato status to activity maniac in one giant leap. Television shows like "The Biggest Loser" promote this image. What often follows sudden surges in physical activity is an ankle sprain, a knee strain, a torn ligament, or a shoulder or back injury. The structural weakness may have been lying dormant, and then became active with sudden extreme activity. Those injuries result in unfortunate delays, which block our intention to become more active.

Some forms of activity, such as Qi Gong and Tai Chi, are especially good for improving coordination and balance in older adults without being overly stressful or likely to strain joints or muscles. These activities work on many levels to support a healthy body-mind-spirit Rhythm.

KEY THINGS TO BE MINDFUL OF BEFORE STRENUOUS PHYSICAL ACTIVITIES

Before taking on strenuous physical activity, make sure that the following cautions are well in place.

1. Avoid getting dehydrated. Be sure to drink plenty of water. As little as 2 percent dehydration can affect athletic performance. If your activity has you sweating, then you need to replace the salt and electrolytes you lose, as well as the water. If you are low in minerals and salt, you can become lightheaded or dizzy easily, even if you are drinking a lot of water.

Sometimes people make the mistake of only drinking water, and actually creating a bigger electrolyte imbalance. In fact, drinking just water when you are sweating a lot will actually further *dilute* the electrolytes in your body and create a greater deficiency! So what you need to do is:

2. Replace electrolytes. There are many ways to replace the electrolytes lost from sweating. You can buy electrolyte packs to add to your drinking water. Or use a premade electrolyte drink. Or you can make your own electrolyte replacement solution:

ESSENTIAL SELF-CARE WHEN DOING STRENUOUS PHYSICAL ACTIVITY

Water—drink plenty of it.

✦

Electrolytes—replace what you lost by sweating (use pre-made or make your own drink)

✦

Start small and basic.

✦

Have fun!

Put a pinch (1/2 teaspoon) of sea salt, a pinch of potassium (either a tablet, or a mashed banana, or Morton's salt substitute), a squeeze of lemon, and a teaspoon of sugar or maple syrup, and mix into a quart of water. This dehydration solution is used in India to successfully treat people with cholera, a condition that results in water- and electrolyte-loss through massive diarrhea.

3. Don't overdo it. Be aware of warning signs such as pain. Don't over-extend joints, and avoid repetitive-stress injuries by stopping at the first sign of strain. Start with small and basic moves before moving to more complicated ones. Learn to feel the difference between good and bad pain—burning in the belly muscle is healthy; sharp pain in the joints is not. Overtraining can occur when exercise is carried on too hard and too long.

Some conditions deserve special care. If you have adrenal fatigue, you need to be extremely cautious with exercise. Check with your doctor first to see if you are ready to start exercising. Too much physical activity can be draining and result in making you feel worse. For some people with adrenal fatigue, standing for five or ten minutes is all they can tolerate. If you can tolerate walking, start off with five minutes or fewer of walking.

Increase the amount very slowly. Your goal is to move only as much as you can tolerate. If you are exhausted afterwards and need to rest later that day or even longer because of the amount of activity you did, you are doing too much. You need to reduce the amount until you find a level that is not exhausting but sustainable.

THE KEY TO VITALIZING YOUR BODY IS TO KEEP IT FUN!

I once bought myself a Nordic Trak—a machine that replicated cross-country skiing. I thought it would help me exercise more. It became the most expensive hat rack I ever had. I never once used it. My point is: everyone is different, and each of us needs to explore the possibilities for activity for ourselves.

Experiment: try different things to help determine what you find enjoyable. Some people do better with a class. Being with a group motivates them to do the activity. Committing to a class helps them muster what they need to continue to show up. Others have no problem spending time alone, whether walking, in their home gym, or following along with a video.

Take a Walk

I am fortunate to have a dog that insists on two walks a day. I have learned that if I dress appropriately, I can feel cozy and comfortably warm and enjoy walking in rain, wind, or snow, as well as in temperatures below freezing. Someone once said, "There is no such thing as bad weather [for walking]; there is just unsuitable clothing." Or, as Thomas A. Clark said in his book, *In Praise of Walking*: "When I spend the day talking I feel exhausted; when I spend it walking I am pleasantly tired."

What do I do on my daily walks? My walks have become as essential as meals for maintaining my sense of wellbeing. Sometimes I bring my cell phone and make it a time for a long, uninterrupted, heart-to-heart conversation with a friend. Often, though, I leave the phone at home, preferring not to be interrupted in my sojourn. I make sure that I am dressed for the weather, so that I get neither chilled or overheated. I wear layers that I can tie around my waist or stuff in my pockets, if they are not needed. Sometimes I bring a small pair of binoculars to focus on the many birds and occasional deer or muskrat I might run across. (Inevitably, the most unusual bird sightings happen when I have forgotten my binoculars—some sort of Murphy's Law.)

As I walk, I frequently remind myself to return to the posture that my Rolfer (Rolfing is a specific form of bodywork) has taught me: chest high, shoulders relaxed, and head up. *Posture has such a powerful effect on emotional tone.* Walking while gazing down at the ground can reinforce a "down" mood, whereas looking straight ahead with head held high can *uplift* a mood. Like many women, I unconsciously hold my neck pitched forward, with my head bent slightly downward. This posture creates a "Dowager's hump" that can become prominent and disfiguring in later life. My Rolfer thinks that this is a posture of deference that women take unconsciously and which reflects their submissive social position relative to men in our society. I have noticed how much more powerful and grounded I feel when I walk or stand with my chest high, neck erect, and head balanced on top. And all I've done is slightly changed my posture!

While walking, I sometimes integrate practices that I learned in yoga class. I take deep belly-breaths, and I consciously relax my shoulders, jaw, brow, and other places that tend to fall into habitual constriction. I also try out different paces. Some days, a fast pace feels good, while on other days a slower, more meandering one suits me better.

Many different traditions endorse walking as a form of meditation. You walk—and when you notice a thought that occurs, consciously release the thought, repeating this process over and over until the mind empties and becomes still.

My walks give me an opportunity to connect with the natural world around me. I smell the variety of smells that change with the seasons. I listen to the sounds of life around me: the various bird songs—the crows that loudly announce my presence, or a nearby hawk—and the music of the pines when the wind catches in their branches. So much is happening. I feel the wind, the moisture in the air, the sound of rain on fallen leaves in autumn. How white and sharp the winter sunlight feels, compared to summer's yellow glow.

I notice the changes that each season brings to all that's around me. I watch as the tree leaves turn colors and fall, drifting lazily down. Sometimes a storm in the night has ripped away all the remaining leaves and the trees stand bare—each with its own unique skeletal form. I marvel at the crystal magic of frost transforming the landscape into fields of diamonds and prisms of light. I breathe in the deep rest of winter and the hush of new- fallen snow. And then there's the excitement of spring, as new green shoots push up out of the dry grass and buds begin to swell on the trees. The incredible parade of flowers, organized so that each plant has its moment of glory as spring opens into summer. Each day is a new adventure.

Take Time-Outs in Nature

We know that fresh air is vitally important for children. The same is true for older folks, too. There is something deeply invigorating about being in nature. The Japanese have a term *shin rin yoku*, which means "forest bathing." Anyone who has been in a forest knows this experience. The Japanese even have a specific word for the light that is filtered through the trees' leaves. How beautifully their language reflects a heightened sense of awareness of nature and how it affects us!

When I visited England, I was amazed to learn about the footpath system they have established that literally makes it possible for one to walk anywhere throughout the entire country. Walking has always been a beloved pastime of the British. When laws about private property and fences began to be established, the people in England passed a law to ensure that they would never be barred from walking over their glorious and beloved hills and valleys. Today, the farmers are obliged to keep a mowed footpath through their fields, and every fence has stiles or gates along the footpath so that people can easily move from field to field without the farmer losing any livestock.

In the United States, unfortunately, "No Trespassing" signs keep us from stepping on privately owned land. Even in the more rural countryside, many roads have enough traffic and little shoulder room, so that walking becomes a dangerous proposition. As a result, unless we drive to a public park to walk, we have little opportunity to walk in a natural setting. Perhaps if we as a nation spent more time in nature, we would have a greater sense of connection with it and a stronger commitment to guard and support the wellbeing of the land around us.

THE RHYTHM OF WORK AND PLAY

Remember the saying, "All work and no play makes Jack a dull boy"? There is a *Rhythm of work and play*. Both work and play are important in a vital, balanced life, but we have neglected our need to play. The question we must ask ourselves is not, "How do I find the time for exercise?" but "Have I created enough *play* in my life?"

There is a dance, a *Rhythm*, of Work and Play—and as a culture, we've lost that awareness. In tribal cultures, when there's work, people do it, often together. But when there's not, people sit around and talk, laugh, or are simply quiet together. They're *enjoying being.* In the movie, "Babies," these kinds of cultural differences were striking. The movie follows four babies—American, Japanese, Mongolian, and African—through their first year of life. The American and Japanese mothers had planned group activities to do with their babies—such as listening to music or strollering. They seemed contrived, disjointed, and not very joyful. In sharp contrast, the African mother seemed to be always laughing, smiling, talking with friends, braiding someone's hair, and enjoying herself with other people, while her baby was crawling around over people or being jiggled around by older children. In one scene, the African mothers were grinding something with a mortar and pestle, and the babies were given two stones to hit together, as babies that age like to imitate what adults are doing. The scenes were joyful.

Some General Exercise Guidelines

There are many ways to incorporate exercise into our lives on a daily basis. Spend time with friends who already enjoy being active. As I mentioned before, take the stairs instead of the elevator; walk up and down the escalators; and park farther away from your destination so you can walk a little more. Instead of eating lunch at your desk, take time on your lunch hour to walk or engage in some form of physical activity.

"How much exercise should I get?" my patients ask. Former U.S. Surgeon General Dr. Vivek H. Murthy announced that research studies found walking 22 minutes a day improved cardiovascular and blood-sugar health significantly. He urged all Americans to undertake a daily brisk walk. If you like to window shop, lock your wallet in the car and give yourself 22 minutes to walk through some shops.

Here are some parameters to keep in mind:

1. Start slow, and increase the time and degree of difficulty gradually, as tolerated.

2. Pick activities and locations that you enjoy.
3. Play around and experiment with new types of activity.
4. Make sure your health supports getting more active by getting a checkup before starting.
5. Resolve any biodynamic structural problems before starting strenuous exercise, to avoid an injury.
6. Listen to your body, and stop when it says to stop.
7. Commit to a daily physical activity of your choice for 28 days—long enough to make it a habit.

REMEMBER TO ENJOY YOURSELF!

Moving is an opportunity to reconnect with the inner child in you that loves to play. Choose a physical activity that brings you more fully present in the moment. Feel your aliveness in motion. Experience gratitude for the body that provides you the opportunity to move joyously with the Rhythm of Life.

⌐∽

CHAPTER FIVE

EMOTION

The Mind-Body Connection

"Mental health is not a destination but a process. It's about how you drive,
not where you are going."
— NOAM SHPANCER, *The Good Psychologist*

EMOTIONS ARE ENERGY IN MOTION

The Rhythm of Emotion is like the wind: ever-changing and sometimes unpredictable. We human beings experience many different
emotions during the course of a single day. These emotions affect not only
our emotional wellbeing but also our physical health. The mind and the
body are intrinsically interconnected.

Most people are already aware of this body-mind connection. Our
language has many common sayings that acknowledge this awareness. We
speak about our intuition as a *gut feeling*. We have a *sensation of butterflies
in our stomach* when we are excited or nervous, and feel *sucker-punched* by
an unpleasant surprise. We say *we feel it in our bones* to describe a certain way of knowing. These and many more commonly used expressions
acknowledge our understanding of a body-mind connection.

A HOLISTIC PERSPECTIVE ON DEPRESSION

"Doctor, I'm so depressed," Madeline told me, her words echoed in her
resigned expression and the flatness in her voice. "I've tried different antidepressant medications but they just make me feel numb. I want to try a

more holistic approach. Can you help me?" A successful businesswoman in her forties, she was smartly dressed and looked trim and fit.

"I'd be glad to," I began. "However," I cautioned, feeling it was important to explain a little about my holistic approach to depression, "contrary to what drug ads would have you think, everyone's depression is *not the same*. This means that the *resolution* of their depression is also unique. So before I can make any recommendations, I need to know a lot more about what depression is like for *you*."

She nodded her agreement. In fact, she looked a bit relieved to hear that I would be finding out more about *her*, rather than inserting her case into some general "treatment template."

So I asked her, "How does your behavior change when you are depressed? What would a fly on the wall observe that is different, when you are depressed?"

Madeline took a deep breath. "Well," she began, "I just can't seem to get going. I'd rather lie in bed and sleep—which makes it hard to keep up with my business."

I nodded in commiseration. "Some people feel like sleeping a lot when they're depressed. Other people have a lot of difficulty sleeping when they're depressed. We're all different, and so depression shows up differently for each of us."

Madeline nodded again. I could see that she was following our conversation with curiosity.

> *We're all different, and so depression shows up*
> *differently for each of us.*

"When you're depressed, how does it affect your appetite and sexuality?" I continued.

"I eat all the time, even when I'm not hungry. And sex—forget it! I don't have any desire, and the overeating makes me feel bad about my body. I feel unattractive."

"What about physical activity?" I pursued further. "How does your depression affect that?"

"When I'm depressed, I stop going to the gym or doing any exercise, which only makes me feel worse." Madeline sounded even more resigned.

"This is helpful information," I told her. "And I have a lot more questions to help me understand your depression better."

Receiving her nod as a go-ahead signal, I asked her a series of questions:

- "Is there a place in your body where your depression seems to be located?"
- "Does it have a particular color or shape?"
- "What does it feel like?"

And, very importantly:

- "When did it begin, and what was going on in your life around that time or just prior to that?"

After asking each question, I paused to hear her response. Some clinicians might fall into the more Western-medical practice of asking only a few questions ("How are you sleeping? How is your appetite?") and then dispensing medication. But for me as a holistic doctor, it's vital to take the time to listen to the patient's *whole* story. Some people have never had the opportunity to tell their whole story before, as a number of my patients have told me after our initial visit together.

What I learn from this deeper listening is how each person's depression really *is* unique. For some, depression feels like they want to sleep all the time. Others can't sleep. Some want to eat a lot; others lose all interest in food. Some can't think, and others can't *stop* thinking. Some cry a lot, some shop a lot, and some are actually very angry.

For some, their depression is part of a down-cycle that began after an extremely arduous up-cycle of work or emotional stress, or both. Maybe the depression is part of adrenal fatigue or exhaustion that has developed slowly over years. For another person, their depression occurred after a great loss or a deep shock, so it has a large *grief* component at the core.

Fear, sadness, and grief are some of the emotions that are found in the shady and dark eddies of our psyche. They live in the Yin part of our nature—the part that is passive rather than active, deep rather than on the surface, diffuse rather than focused. We contain both Yin and Yang qualities. However, our culture sees depression as something to "get over," like the chickenpox. We are told to "suck it up," "get on with it," and "stop navel-gazing."

We do not *want* to feel sad, or mad, or scared, or shame. Yet we all do—*all* of us feel those emotions at times. Our energy and our emotions oscillate, just as energy does in all living things. Sometimes we are up and feeling joy, pleasure, happiness, even ecstasy. At other times we are down and feeling sadness, emptiness, loneliness, hopelessness, grief, anger, or fear.

> *Our culture sees depression as something to "get over," like the chickenpox. Yet our emotions oscillate, just as energy does in all living systems.*

We oscillate like a sine wave, with emotions going up and down—throughout our day and throughout our life. When we accept our own mood oscillations as well as those of others, we de-pathologize sadness and some of the other emotions, such as fear and shame.

The Down Side of Antidepressants

Television ads are full of the latest pharmaceuticals for depression. Current conventional medical practice tends to offer a "one-shoe-fits-all" solution for depression. Feeling blue? Take Prozac!

But, as Madeline informed me, "I've taken antidepressants for years and I'm *still* not sure whether it is actually helping. I'd like to stop taking them."

Many patients have told me that they would like to stop the antidepressants. They feel the antidepressants may have taken the edge off their depression—but, they notice, the trade-off is that *all* their emotions are flat or damped down. Although their grief or despair is less painful when they are on medication, they also don't experience much joy or excitement. And the libido-dampening effect of antidepressants is well known and can make life more difficult in other realms.

Madeline shook her head. "Why can't I just get over it?" she wanted to know.

"That's what the pharmaceutical industry wants you to think their drugs will accomplish," I responded. "Our culture sees states of mind such as depression and sadness as disagreeable and to be shunned. We have no patience or compassion for these moods."

SOME HOLISTIC TREATMENTS FOR DEPRESSION

"What can help me feel less depressed?" Tears appeared ready to spring out of Madeline's eyes.

"I have found that a number of different things help," I began.

Posture

"Sometimes something as simple as changing your *posture* makes a big difference. If you tend to walk looking down at the ground, try consciously *looking up* when you walk. It can create a different mood. This is something I have found helpful for myself, as well."

Nature

Remember *shin rin yoku*, the Japanese word for "forest bathing"? Time spent in nature can be a tremendous mood-lifter. Wise folks who speak about "needing a breath of fresh air" and "clearing the air" are speaking from experience.

Vitamin D

"It's important that we check your Vitamin D levels," I continued. "A number of my patients turned out to have very low Vitamin D3 levels. Some of them found that their mood improved considerably after supplementing with adequate amounts of Vitamin D3."

If a person's Vitamin D level is below the normal range, I recommend that they take 5,000 IU of D3 daily for a month, and then continue with a daily maintenance dose of 2,000-5,000 IU. It is important to take Vitamin D3 *with food*, as it is a fat-soluble vitamin and is best absorbed when the digestion is activated at the end of a meal. Spending time in the sun without sunscreen will enhance your Vitamin D3, as well.

Why are we finding so many people with low Vitamin D? Besides farmers (who comprise less than 1 percent of the population today), most people do not spend enough time in the sun for their bodies to make adequate amounts of Vitamin D. Most windows today are treated to screen out UVB light, which is the spectrum of light that is needed for the body to convert Vitamin D2 into the active form, D3. Even those people who spend at least an hour a day outdoors may not benefit if most of their skin is covered with clothing during that time. Sunscreen will also block UVB.

Boosting Neurotransmitters

"Another factor that can contribute to mood difficulties," I suggested to Madeline, "is a deficiency or imbalance of *neurotransmitters*. There are many good tests available to check neurotransmitter levels, their precursors, or breakdown products."

Madeline frowned in concentration. "Are there natural ways to help that?"

"Yes, there are a lot of possibilities. I have found that supplements such as 5-Hydroxytryptophan, L-Tyrosine, SAM-e, or GABA may be helpful. They provide additional precursors for the neurotransmitters. Then the body is able to make additional quantities, if it needs to."

SOME TREATMENTS FOR DEPRESSION:

Posture changes—look up rather than down when you walk.

Vitamin D—have your levels checked. Your mood may improve with adequate Vitamin D3.

Neurotransmitters—have them checked for deficiencies or imbalances (supplements such as 5-Hydroxytryptophan, L-Tyrosine, SAM-e, or GABA may be helpful).

Lithium in minute amounts may be helpful.

Eliminating sugar and white flour from your diet may lift your mood.

Lithium

"For some people," I continued, "minute amounts of the mineral *lithium* has been helpful for mood problems."

"Isn't lithium what they give people who are bipolar?" Madeline questioned me.

"Yes, lithium has long been used in psychiatry as an effective drug treatment for bipolar disorder. Typical lithium treatment uses doses of 300mg per day and higher. However, those dosages create a lot of side effects, such as interfering with thyroid function and causing significant weight gain. I have found that taking as little as 5 milligrams of lithium a day (one sixtieth the minimum pharmaceutical dose) can be enough to improve some people's depressions. And at that strength, one avoids the unpleasant side effects of large doses of lithium."

Mood-Lifters—Dietary

I added, "For some people, taking sugar and white flour out of the diet (if that is a major component of their diet) can result in an improvement in mood."

Testing

"Because everyone's depression is unique, what they *need* is unique. We may need to test and try a few different possibilities before we find what works best for you." I wanted Madeline to know that she was on a healing journey, and that I was committed to accompany her as long as needed. "I think we also should check your thyroid and adrenal functions."

Together, Madeline and I reviewed the possible steps she could take. We decided to test her Vitamin D3 levels, and check her thyroid and adrenals as well. We also wrote up a schedule to slowly decrease her Prozac dosage and add some 5HTP as she tapered off the medication. She left the office looking less tense, and with a bottle of Rescue Remedy in her hand.

> *Because everyone's depression is unique,*
> *what they need is unique.*

Other organic causes for depression can be a thyroid functioning in the low-normal range, or an underlying adrenal fatigue that needs to be addressed. (You will find more detailed information about the thyroid and adrenals in Chapter Nine: Fatigue and Recovery.)

Additional Tools for Dealing with Depression

It is helpful to find an experienced holistic practitioner who can sort through your story and provide feedback, reflection, and advice. There may be factors that might be contributing to your current mood or state of mind, such as chemical imbalances or vitamin deficiencies, which can be addressed. Other people find that their depression is helped with homeopathy or acupuncture.

The most basic message I would like to convey is: *there is hope.* There is every reason to hope that improvement, if not resolution, can occur.

Deaths, loss, and change are an intrinsic part of the Rhythms of Life. Sometimes, depression is the appropriate response to one's life situation. Chronic pain or disability can be extremely disconcerting and frustrating, at times. Many people have difficulties with family members. Some changes leave us devastated, sad, and depressed.

THE MIND-BODY AND BODY-MIND CONNECTION

We can thank Dr. Candace Pert for providing the scientific proof of the connection between the mind and the body. In 1974, while working in a Johns Hopkins laboratory, she discovered the opioid receptor in the brain. This receptor is the cellular binding site for endorphins—opioid-like substances made in our own bodies.

Scientists had already known about endorphins and other neurotransmitters, such as epinephrine, norepinephrine, serotonin, and dopamine. But they had not been able to determine how they communicated. Each neurotransmitter has a unique effect on the nervous system, as well as on many other systems and parts of the body.

The discovery of the endorphin receptor led to further research, and to the astonishing discovery that neurotransmitter receptor sites existed not only in the brain but in the gut, as well. It had been assumed, prior to that time, that neurotransmitters only communicated with the brain. The image that the "feeling mind" existed only in the brain, separate from the body, could no longer be supported—even from a Western scientific perspective.

Dr. Pert discovered that, in fact, there are more neurotransmitter receptor sites in the gut than in the brain. Based on her own scientific discoveries, Dr. Pert became a leading figure in the growing holistic health movement. Her book, *Molecules of Emotion*, is a fascinating look at the evolution of her own thinking as well as a peek into the world of academic science (and its politics). In the wake of her discoveries, the scientific field of psychoneuroimmunology (PNI) has developed to study the mind-body connection. PNI takes an interdisciplinary approach, incorporating psychology, neuroscience, immunology, physiology, genetics, pharmacology, molecular biology, psychiatry, behavioral medicine, infectious diseases, endocrinology, and rheumatology.

> *The image that the "feeling mind" existed only in the brain, separate from the body, could no longer be supported—even from a Western scientific perspective.*

THERAPIES BASED ON THE MIND-BODY CONNECTION

Many new modes of therapy using the mind-body connection have evolved to facilitate work with emotional issues and trauma. Some of them begin with the *mind*, using words to explain the situation, then expanding to working with the *body* for healing and resolution. Some of these therapies include Cognitive Behavioral Therapy (CBT), Gestalt, psychodrama, Hellinger work, ShadowWork, dance therapy, and more.

Other therapeutic modalities start by addressing the physical-symptom presentation, then proceed to include the emotional—using the *body-mind* rather than the mind-body approach. These approaches include various myofascial therapies such as Somatic Experiencing, Rolfing, Feldenkreis, Alexander, Cranial Osteopathy, Cranio-Sacral therapy, Yoga Therapy, and other physical modalities that include touch.

What underlies this gamut of approaches is the fact that emotions are *not* just thoughts in our brains. They actually *live* as energetic patterns in our bodies. These emotions are physically stored in the collagen. Collagen is the key; it is the building block of many different types of tissue, including nerves, muscles, fascia, bone, and blood. It is also the connective-tissue material that interfaces and interconnects our entire body.

Collagen has a triple helical piezoelectric structure. ("Piezoelectric" means that it is capable of creating an electrical charge and being a force field.) The helical structure of collagen is crystal-like. Stresses such as physical trauma deform the crystal. These deformations can remain in the tissues, buried and forgotten until the exact right touch succeeds in releasing them. At the moment of release there can be symptoms of an autonomic-nervous-system discharge, such as shaking, twitching, goose bumps, sweating, and even crying. There may or may not also be a recognizable emotional release that accompanies the collagen-restructuring effect. A trained and skillful body worker will recognize these symptoms as the release of trauma that may have been held in the collagen for years, or even decades.

Several massage therapists and physical therapists I have spoken with have witnessed emotional releases in their clients during a massage or physical-therapy treatment session. These releases may be vocal or physical—sometimes shaking, or laughter or tears. I knew one physical therapist who insisted that her clients bring their psychotherapists with them to her physical therapy sessions to facilitate processing any emotions that were released during her work.

Holistic Treatments for Anxiety

"My problem is anxiety," said Colleen at our first appointment. "I'd like to find a holistic approach that helps me."

Colleen was a young-looking woman in her thirties, dressed in layers of drab-colored clothing. She sat quietly, appearing rather drawn into herself. Her eyes darted out occasionally to get a quick look at me.

Anxiety is perhaps the most common complaint I hear in my office besides fatigue. *Generalized Anxiety Disorder* (GAD) is the medical term for it, and it is so widespread today that it could be considered an epidemic. Its hallmark is excessive, out-of-control worry. The origins or causes of anxiety seem to be quite complex and can include a familial tendency and genetic factors, as well as environmental influences. Environmental influences can include specific job or occupation factors, home life, and dietary habits. As a holistic doctor, I need to take all these influences into consideration.

Colleen looked at me despairingly. "Have you found anything to help anxiety? I really need help!"

"Oh, yes," I responded, wanting to sound reassuring. "I have found many different approaches to be helpful for anxiety. Although Western medicine has lumped everyone's experience under the diagnosis of 'anxiety,' I see it differently. As a holistic doctor, my view is that *we are all unique individuals, and we each have our own unique anxiety.*"

I saw that I had Colleen's attention now. "Tell me more about your anxiety," I continued. And I asked her a lot of questions: "When did it start?" "What are the specific physical sensations that accompany your anxiety?" "Where in your body do you feel them?" "What seems to make it better? What seems to make it worse?" "Are there specific thoughts that seem to accompany the physical sensations?"

She answered thoughtfully; and as I listened to her responses to these and other questions, I began to understand more deeply what she meant by her "anxiety." Our conversation also helped me determine which interventions would be most helpful for her.

Panic Attacks

"Do you ever have panic attacks?" I asked Colleen.

"I think so. I've made several trips to the Emergency Room because I was scared I might be having a heart attack," she replied.

"What was going on for you at that time?" I wanted to hear her own experience, what her body sensations were, and how she responded to them.

"There was pressure in my chest," she reported, "and I felt a tingling—almost numbness—in my arms. I felt like I couldn't take a deep breath, and my heart was pounding. I was scared to death!"

Every day, people having a panic attack wind up in the emergency room because they think they are having a heart attack or some other extreme medical condition. *Fear* is the overriding emotion experienced during a panic attack, and fear itself can produce many of these kinds of symptoms (e.g., shallow breathing, pounding heart).

I also wanted to make sure that what Colleen had experienced did not indicate some physiological problem, such as a heart condition. "What happened when you got to the ER?" I asked.

"The emergency room doctor checked everything out and couldn't find anything wrong." Colleen added, "They told me I was having a panic attack and to go home and see my own doctor. When I did, she gave me anti-anxiety medication—but the side effects made me feel worse. And when the medication wore off, my anxiety was worse than ever. I finally got off the medication, but I still have anxiety."

"Do you tend to avoid places where there might be a lot of people?" was my next question.

"Yes," she replied, looking at me a little quizzically, as if wondering how I might have known this. "I go food shopping late at night," she confided, "because there are very few people in the store then."

I asked her this because over time, the *anticipatory fear* of having a panic attack can cause people to avoid settings where a previous panic attack occurred. People who experience panic attacks may start to avoid crowds. Their circle of activity gets smaller and smaller, and they slowly withdraw from social life.

If the panic attacks continue, the sufferer becomes more and more afraid to go anywhere and becomes a virtual prisoner in his or her own home. *Agoraphobia*, a fear of going into new or public places, can become a real problem for these people, creating many difficulties in their ability to carry on a full life. According to Wikipedia, about 3.2 million American adults between 18 and 54 suffer from agoraphobia.

A Diet to Reduce Anxiety

Diet can play a part in emotional imbalances such as anxiety. As the rapper Danny Brown said in a recent NPR interview, referring to his own past experiences of anxiety and depression: "If you start livin' unhealthy, you start thinkin' unhealthy."

I turned to Colleen and suggested, "Let's take a look at your food diary." She pulled out her phone, where she had carefully logged all the food she had eaten the previous week. I noticed that she had consumed a lot of fast foods and soda, as well as caffeine and refined-flour products such as bread, cereal, and pasta.

"A good first step would be to eliminate specific foods that are well known to stimulate the nervous system." I clarified further, "That would include stimulants such as coffee, caffeinated teas, chocolate, sugar, and energy drinks; and to avoid any products that contain guarana, gambogia, or caffeine."

"That makes sense to me," Colleen nodded in agreement. "I can do that."

Since she was agreeable, I decided to venture further and provide more information, "I've also had a number of patients report that their anxiety decreased after they eliminated wheat and wheat products from their diet."

Colleen was busy taking notes.

"So," I went on, "you might want to avoid any wheat during the next month and see if it makes a difference in your anxiety level."

She nodded again.

I added, "Some people have noticed a decrease in their anxiety when they increased the amount of healthy-sourced saturated fat in their diet."

Colleen looked surprised. "Fat! But I thought that fat was bad for you!"

I explained, "Our nerve cells, or neurons, are enclosed in a myelin sheath. This myelin sheath serves to insulate the nerve cells, like the insulation on an electrical wire. We are all familiar with the dangers of a frayed or poorly insulated electric cord. Electrical shocks and short-outs, even fires, can result from faulty insulation. A well-functioning myelin sheath is key to a healthy nervous system."

"And where do fats come in?" Colleen wanted to know.

"Saturated fats break down into fatty acids, the building blocks of the myelin sheath. Adequate fats in the diet can improve the function of the nervous system—in part because the nerve cells are better insulated. Increasing the amount of good fat in the diet can be extremely helpful for people with anxiety whose diet has been low in saturated fat."

ANXIETY-REDUCING DIET:

Eliminate foods that stimulate the nervous system, especially stimulants (e.g., coffee, caffeinated teas, chocolate, sugar, energy drinks, etc.).

Eliminate wheat and wheat products for a month to see effects on anxiety level.

Increase healthy saturated fats

"And all this time I've been avoiding fat, thinking it was bad for me!" Colleen exclaimed.

"You're not alone in thinking that," I agreed with her. "But doctors at Johns Hopkins found that a diet composed of mostly saturated fats helped children with epilepsy when medication didn't work. The ketogenic diet has been in use since 1922 to help infants and children with refractory epileptic seizures that are difficult to control with medication. The Mayo Clinic and Johns Hopkins hospital have conducted research confirming the benefits."

The classic ketogenic diet contains a 4:1 ratio by weight of fat to combined protein and carbohydrate. The saturated fats used include: coconut oil; palm oil; lard; suet; and chicken, goose, and duck fat. This diet has been very successful in reducing or eliminating seizure problems, and illustrates the positive effects of saturated fats on the nervous system. (More details on the benefits of saturated fats can be found in the chapter on Nutrition.)

"I'll give this diet a try," Colleen promised before leaving my office. "After all, what do I have to lose?"

Anxious Thoughts

By the time of her next appointment, Colleen reported that her anxiety had decreased considerably after eliminating caffeine and other stimulants, and she was sleeping better. She had also increased the amount of fat in her diet and stopped using low-fat products.

"That's really good news!" I beamed. "Good for you!" And we celebrated silently for a moment.

But there was another matter that concerned her. "Sometimes I can't seem to control my thoughts," she told me.

"Are there any specific thoughts that keep repeating?"

"Yes, sometimes it feels like an endless loop!"

Flower Essence Remedies

"I have a suggestion," I said. "There is a remedy specifically for repetitive thoughts in the *Bach flower remedies*. They help reduce the persistence of such thoughts." (The Appendix at the back of this book lists the Bach flower remedies and the associated thought patterns that they address.)

"You may be familiar with Rescue Remedy?" I asked.

Colleen looked puzzled.

I continued, "It's a well-known mixture of five Bach flower remedies that can be very helpful when you feel ungrounded or have sustained a shock. I usually carry a dropper bottle of Rescue Remedy in my purse. "

As with all the flower remedies, to use them you put four drops in your mouth every fifteen minutes, for as often as it is needed. Another method is to put four drops in your water bottle so you get a dose with each sip of water.

"What do you think?" I asked Colleen. "Would you be willing to try using flower essences to see if they are helpful?"

She had never heard of flower essence remedies before, and although she seemed a little doubtful, she nodded and said, "Sure, let's give it a try." Together, we chose those Bach flowers that correlated with her specific thought patterns, and I made up a mixture for her in a small dropper bottle.

"You could take the first dose now, while you're still in my office," I suggested. "Some of my patients who did so found that their anxiety decreased by 50 percent or more within ten minutes of taking the drops."

She squeezed four drops of the remedy into her mouth right then and there.

I have found Bach flower remedies to be powerful helpers in the realm of emotional health, although science has not advanced to the point of being able to explain *why* they and other flower essences work. The full range of Bach Flower remedies is available in many health-food stores, as are a number of other flower remedy collections that have been developed. Although I haven't used these others as much, I have heard good reports of their effectiveness from other practitioners.

"How are you feeling now?" I inquired after ten or more minutes had passed since she had taken the drops.

Colleen looked a bit surprised, "I feel less anxious, and my thoughts seemed to have calmed down." She appeared visibly more relaxed, and left eager to continue with the flower essence.

When she returned for her next appointment, she reported, "I'm feeling much better. There's less anxiety and I'm sleeping better. The drops seem to work pretty well."

"Great," I said. "Why don't you continue using them until our next appointment, and we'll see how you're doing at that point."

Essential Oils

Colleen had another question. "My sister has been learning about essential oils, and she wants me to try some. She thinks they can help my mood. What do you think?"

"Essential oils can be used for a great many health conditions, including depression and anxiety," I responded. "I use some myself, but I don't consider myself an expert on them. However, I see no harm in trying them to see if they help you."

Essential oils have long been known to have powerful effects on mood. Perfumers and soap makers have known this and used scents for thousands of years to great advantage. The scent of *lavender* can create a sense of gentle wellbeing and relaxation. *Rose* has long been touted as the scent of love. *Patchouli* is known for its spicy stimulation, and *eucalyptus* for its deeply penetrating, muscle-relaxing heat.

Smells, via olfactory nerve input, bypass the frontal brain and connect directly with the limbic system, which is the seat of the emotions. Smells can trigger emotions as well as memories. Many essential oil companies create specific blends to enhance or disperse certain moods or states of mind. If you have trouble finding essential oils locally, the Internet can provide a list of companies that sell them. I have used many different companies' oils, and especially like MZ Alchemist Oils and blends formulated by Mikael Zayat.

I once had the opportunity to sit with a great storyteller from India who was also a maker of essential oils and had crafted many of his own unique oil blends. As he told us a story, he would add different essential oils to a diffuser next to him. The effect of these diffused oils was to create a three-dimensional experience of the story while he told it. At different times we smelled the cave, the meadow, the forest, and more. It was truly magical.

EMDR (Eye Movement Desensitization and Reprocessing)

"Besides essential oils," Colleen wanted to know, "what else can help anxiety?"

"Have you heard of EMDR?" I asked her.

"No, what's that?" she replied.

"EMDR, or Eye Movement Desensitization and Reprocessing, is a specific therapeutic technique that separates the memory of a traumatic event from the *emotions* evoked by the memory. I have had patients who successfully used EMDR to relieve anxiety that had its roots in past trauma."

EMDR has been very helpful with children as well as adults who have post-traumatic distress symptoms. You can find therapists trained in

EMDR by going on the *Psychology Today* therapist directory online and specifying "EMDR": *https://therapists.psychologytoday.com/emdr*

CBT (Cognitive Behavioral Therapy)

"There's also Cognitive Behavioral Therapy, or CBT, which can help decrease panic attacks," I added. "The CBT therapist suggests an action plan that is designed to desensitize the person to their triggers so they develop greater ease in public situations over time."

Colleen was listening intently, so I volunteered more information. "Some of my patients have found CBT to be very helpful. One man could not leave the house without experiencing severe anxiety. In addition, he suffered bouts of diarrhea, which made it impossible for him to eat anything if he needed to leave his house. You can imagine how that limited his life."

"Wow, that sounds awful!" Colleen exclaimed. "At least I'm not *that* bad off!"

"After a year and a half of CBT," I told her, "he was able to leave home without anxiety, and he began to pursue his old interests in horseback riding and art classes. He felt he had succeeded in getting his life back, and he was thrilled." (More information on CBT can be found in the Glossary at the end of this book.)

Over the next months, Colleen's anxiety became less and less of a problem. She continued to eat lots of good saturated fats and avoided stimulants and wheat in her diet. She stopped having panic attacks. Her life expanded and grew richer as she felt able to pursue her many interests both old and new ones. I haven't seen her for a long time now, and assume she is doing well.

Medical Cannabis

We can think more about medical use of cannabis now that (as of 2019) it has been legalized for medical use in 33 states including Maryland, where I practice. Close to 80 million Americans can now legally access various cannabis products in their states. In my experience, some people have found it very helpful for anxiety and sleep issues, particularly the CBD component.

As a side note, I also have patients who found it useful for migraine treatment and pain relief. Several of my patients were able to wean off opiates with cannabis use.

As human beings, we cannot avoid suffering. Yet somehow we continue to hold onto the idea that our life should be one long endless happy ending. And when we don't feel happy, we think we're not okay and we need to *do* something about it to change it.

But what if, maybe, we are experiencing exactly what we need at the moment?

A resource book that I have personally found very helpful is *Swamplands of the Soul: New Life in Dismal Places*, by Dr. James Hollis. Dr. Hollis delves into the many dark emotional states we humans experience, such as Guilt, Grief, Loss, Betrayal, Doubt, Loneliness, Despair, Depression, Obsessions, Addictions, Anger, Fear, Angst, and Anxiety. He offers some guidance on how to retrieve the nugget of gold—the gift—that these dismal places may hold for us. Another helpful resource is the book *The Mood Cure*, by Julia Ross.

Psychotherapy

From time immemorial, people have been comforted and helped by sharing their problems with others. The power of deep listening, of truly being heard, cannot be overemphasized. Finding a trained therapist, one who can accompany you to the darkest places and provide support as you journey back, can be immensely helpful. Many therapists are also trained in mind-body modalities.

Some Mayan Views on Mood Disorders

I once attended a workshop given by Dr. Rosita Arvigo on depression and other mood disorders. Dr. Arvigo spent eleven years in Belize studying, apprenticing, and practicing with a traditional Mayan healer (a *curandero*) and Mayan midwives. Over the years, she came to understand the way the indigenous Mayan culture viewed and treated mental health. The Mayan perspective does not see or treat depression as a single phenomenon, but rather as a number of distinct and different mental/emotional states. Each state has its own cause or cascade of causes, as well as a unique treatment protocol.

One type of depression is called *Invidia*. This emotional state can arise quite suddenly. The symptoms of Invidia include lack of interest in everything, waking with frightening palpitations, bad dreams, bad luck, close calls, shaking hands, and losing things.

Dr. Arvigo explained *Invidia* by telling the story of a young girl, about fifteen years old, who lived in a little village in Mexico. One Saturday in summer, the village held a fiesta and dance, and it happened that the girl's mother was away visiting a relative. The girl decided to wear a new red dress that her cousin in the United States had sent her. That night at the dance, she was the center of all the men's' and boys' attention. She did not notice her girlfriends standing at the edge of the dance floor, watching with fierce eyes and speaking sharp words about her.

The next day, when her mother returned, she found her daughter moody, uninterested in her usual interests, and interacting in mean-spirited ways with her younger sisters and brothers—all very much out of character for her. The mother made inquiries about what had happened while she was gone. On hearing the story of the red dress and the dance, she realized that her daughter was suffering from *Invidia*. The mother sought the help of a curandero; and after she had treated her daughter according to the curandero's instructions, the girl was soon restored to her usual pleasant self.

Another kind of depression that we might call anxiety is exemplified in the fussy and fretful state of a baby after returning home from the market or another crowded public outing. In this case, the baby is thought to be the victim of *mal ojo* or *ojo caliente*. This is the result of too many people gazing on that baby with mixed emotions of desire and covetousness, as well as anger, jealousy, and ill wishes. Wise mothers have learned to use prevention against *mal ojo* and keep their babies covered and out of sight when they go out in public places.

Yet another form of depression is *Pesar*—grief due to loss. It is characterized by deep sighing, sleep problems, palpitations, nightmares, and tortured thoughts about what could or should be.

Susto is a kind of depression consisting of a constant state of flight-or-fight. Sleep is light, and there is underlying anxiety and panic attacks. Chronic indigestion is present. A sudden shock to the system can produce sustained agitation to the nervous system. Dr. Arvigo described the case of a baby who was suddenly jolted awake by a dog and cat fighting under its crib. *Susto* can occur from accidents, war, trauma, abuse, and sudden frights. We can see that *Susto* could be another culture's interpretation of what we call "post-traumatic stress."

Tristessa is *Susto* and *Pesar* that is hidden: sadness and depression for a seemingly unknown reason. It is characterized by tortured and suicidal thoughts and self-blame. The key here is that the causes are unclear to the person experiencing *Tristessa*. Typically, in Belize, in this case one would approach a healer for intervention and help.

These descriptions of *Invidia, Pesar, Ojo Caliente, Susto,* and *Tristessa* broaden our perspective of depression. They describe a multi-faceted, multi-factorial phenomenon. How we view and treat mental/emotional conditions can vary widely, depending on our cultural beliefs and paradigms. Moreover, as we look at the many different healing modalities available, we find that there are many treatment options in addition to pharmaceuticals.

A multicultural, holistic perspective provides a deeper awareness and appreciation for the uniqueness of each person's depression. It would be a grave disservice to simply prescribe an antidepressant without a deeper inquiry into the nature of each person's experience of their depression and the stories surrounding them.

POST TRAUMATIC STRESS DISORDER—PTSD

"I think my son has PTSD," Mrs. Gomez, an older patient of mine, told me at one of her appointments. "Since he came back from the war, he hasn't been the same. The whole family is worried. I think his marriage is in trouble." Her eyes held sadness and grief. "We don't know how to help him!"

Post-Traumatic Stress Disorder, or PTSD, has come into the news and public awareness in recent times, largely due to the number of veterans returning from military service in Iraq and Afghanistan in the second decade of the 21st century. We have been made aware of the high rate of suicide in these returning veterans—twenty-two a day at the time of this writing.

As a physician, I have heard family members of returned veterans speak of the difficulty these veterans experience upon re-entering civilian life after their experiences of war. The military is very good at training warriors for war, but not so skillful in returning warriors to a life of peace in the community. We need a *Re*-Boot Camp at the end of military service.

Post-Traumatic Stress Disorder does not only occur from trauma experienced in war situations. It also can result from childhood abuse, sexual abuse, and other non-military trauma. It is estimated that at least half the population has experienced some kind of deep trauma or abuse. These wounds are not visible. It is important to be aware that we cannot tell *who* may be carrying the burden of PTSD. It could be the fellow driving the car next to us in the traffic jam, or standing behind us in the checkout line, or sitting in the waiting room with us.

> *It is estimated that at least half the population has experienced some kind of deep trauma or abuse. These wounds are not visible.*

"It's important to understand what your son may be experiencing," I told Mrs. Gomez. "Do you know the symptoms of PTSD?"

"Well, I've heard that people may have flashbacks," she began, "and I know he has trouble sleeping because of nightmares."

"Yes, those are common. Sometimes words, objects, sounds, or situations that remind him of the traumatic event can trigger re-experiencing, or *flashbacks*. Re-experiencing symptoms may cause problems in a person's everyday routine. They can even start from the person's own thoughts and feelings."

"He won't go anywhere," Mrs. Gomez went on, "just stays home and keeps to himself. He doesn't want to see his old friends or do any of the things he used to enjoy. It's like he's numb." She shook her head sadly.

"Were you ever in a bad accident?" I asked.

"Oh yes, a car accident several years ago. It was awful!" Her voice became tense as she remembered.

"Did you find it hard to get back to driving again?"

"Yes, I don't think I drove for a while, and it was quite a while before I could relax when I was driving."

I nodded sympathetically. "Things that remind a person of the traumatic event can trigger avoidance behavior and cause a person to change his or her personal routines."

"Yes, as I mentioned, my son hardly goes out of the house, these days,"

"Does he seem on edge a lot?" I inquired.

"Oh yes, he's so tense! He yells at his kids when they get loud or startle him. I think they've become afraid to be around him."

Hyper-arousal symptoms are usually constant, instead of being triggered only by specific things that remind the person of a traumatic event. These symptoms can make the person feel stressed and angry, and may make it hard to do daily tasks such as sleeping, eating, or concentrating.

It's natural to have some of these symptoms after a dangerous event. Sometimes people have very serious symptoms that go away after a few weeks. This is called "Acute Stress Disorder," or ASD. It's when the symptoms last more than a few weeks and become an ongoing problem that they are labeled "PTSD." Some people with PTSD don't show any symptoms for weeks or months, or even years. Some Vietnam veterans found that their PTSD symptoms were triggered by the bombing of the World Trade Center on September 11, 2001—more than *thirty years* after they had returned from war.

What Causes Triggers in PTSD?

The brain is composed of three parts: the forebrain, or neocortex; the midbrain; and the hindbrain. The hindbrain, or Reptilian brain, is the oldest part of the brain. It includes the limbic system, which is involved in memory and the amygdala. The Reptilian brain is concerned with *survival*. Its primary emotions are *fear* and *anger*. The Reptilian brain has no concept of past and present time. Memories held in this part of the brain exist as if happening *now*.

When we find ourselves in a life-threatening situation, the Reptilian brain is activated more than fifty times faster than the forebrain. This activation stimulates a number of physiological responses:

- Blood is preferentially shunted to the heart and lungs, as well as the skeletal muscles.

- Neurotransmitters that stimulate, such as norepinephrine and epinephrine, are released, as well as endorphins to dampen pain sensations.

- Our senses are heightened. We see, hear, smell, and taste more acutely.

- Our peripheral vision expands.

In short, we are in a heightened-awareness state, ready to face the life-threatening force with the three basic instinctual responses: *fight, flight, or freeze.*

Memories of these life-threatening traumatic events are stored in the *amygdala.* Their heightened quality is different from that of *non*-traumatic memories, which are stored in another part of the brain. These traumatic memories include sounds, smells, tastes, touch, and/or visuals. Sounds, smells, tastes, touches, and/or visuals in the present that are similar to the original experience can become a *trigger.* Triggering sets off the fight, flight, or freeze response in the Reptilian brain. Because the amygdala cannot distinguish what has happened in the past from what is happening now, people with PTSD experience a reenactment of the past traumatic experience as if it were happening right now. This is called a *flashback,* because the person is transported back to a past traumatic experience in a flash.

In sum, the rational forebrain is temporarily hijacked by the Reptilian brain.

A fully functioning forebrain can distinguish between a bag of trash on the side of the road in Topeka, Kansas, and a potential explosive device on the side of the road in Iraq. It has the capacity to be logical and judicious and say, "Aw, come on now, we're in Topeka, Kansas, and that's just a bag of trash, not an IED." The problem is that the Reptilian brain's activation is fifty times faster than the forebrain's response time. Moreover, the forebrain only fully matures when a person is about twenty-five years of age. Unfortunately, many military veterans, as well as childhood victims of abuse, experienced their trauma and subsequent re-triggering years before their forebrain became fully functional and able to help them.

When people who suffer from Post-Traumatic Stress Disorder get triggered, the whole psycho-neuro-physiological cascade involved in the fight, flight, or freeze response is set into motion. Some people live in an almost constant state of hyper-arousal. This is not a disease but rather a hijacked repercussion of the normal Reptilian brain's response. Some civilians and military may have lived in a hyper-vigilant, life-or-death state for hours, days, weeks, or months. They may have turned to alcohol and drugs to reduce the intensity of this hyper-arousal state.

Inevitably, some people become addicted to the high endorphin release that occurs in the hyper-stimulated state. Some returning veterans may experience civilian life as flat, boring, and colorless when they are not in a hyper-aroused state. They may feel like they are less alive than when they were in the service. Some of them use thrill-seeking, risk-taking activities such as speeding or reckless driving to raise their adrenalin levels. One of the most common ways that veterans of the Iraq and Afghanistan wars die after returning home is in single-vehicle motorcycle accidents. In desperation for that adrenalin rush, they urge their motorcycle to greater and greater speeds, ultimately losing control of their vehicle and resulting in a fatal accident. Others self-medicate through drugs or alcohol.

Post-Traumatic Stress Disorder is not a new phenomenon; only the name is new. It was coined in the 1980s and put into the DSM-III, the diagnostic guide used to categorize and define psychological conditions. PTSD is only the latest term to be added to the many previous war-time diagnoses, including: "railway spine"; "stress syndrome"; "nostalgia"; "soldier's heart"; "shell shock"; "battle fatigue"; "combat stress reaction"; "or traumatic war neurosis." Some of these terms date back to the nineteenth century, which is indicative of the universal nature of the condition.

Vets Journey Home

"What can we do to help my son?" Mrs. Gomez' voice was almost pleading by now.

"You are asking the million-dollar question," I said. "I wish there were a simple answer. Many different things have been tried with varying success. I have met a number of military veterans suffering from PTSD. Many of them had gone to individual and group therapy at the Veterans Administration and taken medications for years, yet they found little relief of their symptoms."

Mrs. Gomez listened closely. "The medications my son's taking don't seem to be helping," she said, nodding.

I had something else to offer. "I was involved with a weekend program called the Bamboo Bridge," I told her, "started by a Vietnam veteran and a Sergeant Major's daughter in the 1990s. It developed into a program that's now called Vets Journey Home, which I have staffed a number of times. I saw some veterans experience a significant reduction of their PTSD during those weekends. Their lives improved dramatically after participating in the program. And the effects seemed to be long lasting."

I gave Mrs. Gomez a Vets Journey Home brochure, which also listed their website: *www.vetsjourneyhome.org*. She took it gratefully.

Rapid Resolution Therapy

"I have also seen amazing results with hypnosis," I continued. "I have observed one approach in particular—Rapid Resolution Therapy—to be effective for both veterans and civilians in releasing trauma and reducing re-triggering. Dr. John Connolly, who has trained hundreds of hypnotherapists in his technique, developed this approach. And I have had at least one patient who was greatly helped by it."

When I first met Mr. Johnson, a man in his mid-seventies, he was unable to walk without support. He shuffled down the hall on his wife's arm and spoke in a quavering whisper. He looked like someone with advanced neurological impairment.

Mr. Johnson came to see me because he felt he was overmedicated and wanted help sorting out his medications. He was taking a number of different medications prescribed by a number of different doctors. At the time of his first appointment, he was taking three different psychiatric medications. (This seems to be the current fashion in psychiatric pharmacologic treatment—if one drug doesn't help, add a second and then a third.)

Over time, as we slowly decreased his antipsychotic medication, his speech became louder and clearer. Once off that medication entirely, his balance returned and his step became firm. He no longer needed any support while walking.

At the end of one of his appointments, his wife mentioned, "I wish Jim could sleep in bed with me instead of always sleeping in a recliner."

My curiosity was piqued. "Is that right?? I inquired. "You only sleep in a recliner?"

"It's true," Mr. Johnson explained. "I can't go to sleep in a bed, because when I was a child bad things happened when I fell asleep in my bed." He explained that he had been repeatedly molested in his bed after falling asleep. Since then, the only way he could fall asleep was in a chair. And that is how he had slept for many, many years.

I asked him, "Would you *like* to be able to sleep in a bed?"

"Oh yes, definitely," was his immediate response.

I suggested that he see a hypnotist I knew who specialized in Rapid Resolution Therapy.

"And after only one session," I reported now to Mrs. Brown, "he was sleeping soundly in his bed for the first time in many, many years—and continued to do so."

Mrs. Brown's eyes widened upon hearing this story, and I could see a glimmer of hope there. So I looked up the names of Rapid Resolution Therapy practitioners in her son's area. Supported by this information as well as the Vets Journey Home brochure, she looked more hopeful when she left than she had when she'd first come in.

(To find out about Rapid Resolution Therapy, check out this website: *http://www.rapidresolutiontherapy.com.*)

There are many more programs today for the traumatized veteran than even ten years ago as the public's awareness has grown. Some of these newer programs include working with horses, farming, and psychedelic journeys. These programs seem to have good success.

A Word about Psychedelics

> "Among other things, neuroplasticity means that emotions such as happiness and compassion can be cultivated in much the same way that a person can learn through repetition to play golf and basketball or master a musical instrument, and that such practice changes the activity and physical aspects of specific brain areas."
> —ANDREW WEIL, M.D.

Michael Pollan, in his book, *How to Change Your Mind*, describes what he calls our "default mode of consciousness." The default mode is our usual way of thinking, perceiving, and defining ourselves and our world. He details the recent resurgence of scientific studies focusing on psychedelics such as psilocybin, and their success in opening up new neural pathways and expanding our view of life outside of the default mode.

The concept of neural diversity and the success of various psychedelics in treating the anxiety of terminal cancer patients, addiction, and treatment-resistant depression is explored in detail in Pollan's book. These studies are currently being conducted within well-known institutions such as Johns Hopkins University and New York University in the US, and the Imperial College in England. This may be a realm of real hope for many.

GRIEF

> "We must drop, unguarded into the holy bath of grief, inside of which all truly happy men and women must bathe to transform the great losses of life, in war, sicknesses, the loss of homelands and the loss of one's confidence in human decency into a wailing that ends in poetry and elegant praise of the ability to feel. For desire, mistaken for love, without the capacity to truly feel the losses that actual loving entails, is what makes murderers of people who have no home friendly enough to allow them both the complete sadnesses and joys their love can feel."
>
> —MARTIN PRECHTEL, *Stealing Benefacio's Roses*

One of the biggest myths about grief is that we get over it. True heart-breaking grief is a transformative experience. In the grieving process, we are permanently altered. Life goes on and we go on, albeit as our altered self. The heart is broken—broken open—in the process. When the heart breaks open, there is a feeling of vulnerability, of fragility. With grief, we experience its paradoxical essence: the *constant presence of absence*. One lives with the constant presence of the loss; it has energy, and energy is power. The paradox is that although the grief is very palpable in a feeling sense, there is no physical manifestation to tie it to. Sometimes the loss can feel like an amputation.

One of my patients who came from a large, close-knit family called me one day, desperately pleading for help. Her young adult child had been killed in a tragic accident and the funeral was the next day. "How can I face it?" she asked. "I can't pull myself together. Can't you give me something?"

I could feel her suffering—it was overwhelming her. I reassured her that no one *expected* her to be pulled together. That it was totally *appropriate* for her to be overcome with grief and not be able to function in her usual capable manner. I encouraged her to *feel* the grief rather than numb it out. I reassured her that she would not drown in her grief, even though that was her fear in that moment. I also assured her that I would continue to be available to help her and support her. I suggested that she try to live through the next few days without using mind-numbing drugs, which would only delay her from experiencing her emotions. After our conversation, she chose not to use any medication.

Some years later, she thanked me for my support and guidance at that time. She has since found a new balance point and appreciates the many gifts in her life.

Grief can bring us alive more fully. It has a unique journey in each one of us. And the best we can do is honor our process of grieving. Sometimes tears come up and we are overwhelmed with sadness. The best thing to do is just ride the wave of grief—let the tears flow, let the sobs out, let the wails be heard, without judgment. Sometimes people around us are uncomfortable with emotions and will attempt to stop our expression of grief with words of "comfort" and offers of tissues. These ministrations only serve to close down the release of grief that has welled up in that moment. I have suggested that people take a drive to a cemetery, park and just allow the tears and wails to come out. In that setting, no one will feel the need to disturb you and you can continue until you feel complete.

Grief can bring us alive more fully.

If you are in a situation where you cannot express your grief in the moment, promise to give yourself a time and a place in the actual near future when you can release them. It is very important to keep that promise. Emotions are energy. Like other emotions that are not released, they can be stored in the body-memory, in the collagen. The body will store that grief and it may express it later in some physiological problem—a cough or breathing problem; a pain; a difficulty with focusing one's thoughts; the absence of any feeling; or even something like a tumor or a cyst. Remember, the body-mind-spirit are all interconnected.

> *Emotions are energy. Like other emotions that*
> *are not released, they can be stored in the body-*
> *memory, in the collagen. The body will store*
> *that grief and it may express it later in some*
> *physiological problem.*

After my husband of twenty-five years left, I was in shock. Even though our relationship had not been very loving during the previous couple of years, the idea that our marriage would end had not occurred to me. Despite being in shock, my life did not stop. I still had patients who wanted my help, children and grandchildren to attend to, and my friends and community life. My garden needed attention, as did a thousand other things. I journeyed on, living with the constant presence of absence. I thought I was handling my grief well—crying at times, wailing, and writing about it.

However, my body grew a cyst in my ovary, bigger than a grapefruit. A friend who has a machine that can sense cellular imbalances through electromagnetic currents ran her machine on me to determine the cause of the tumor. The machine said it was not cancer, not a virus or bacteria, and not a mineral or vitamin deficiency. The machine said I had an imbalance in the second and fourth chakra. Blockages in the chakras are often influenced by our negative judgments. The judgment that blocks the second-chakra energy is: *My aliveness hurts or kills.* The judgment that blocks the fourth chakra is: *I'm not enough,* or *I'm too much.* Over the course of the next several months, my healing journey included acupuncture, castor-oil packs, affirmations, forgiveness work, homeopathic remedies, and essential oils. It seemed like every minute I wasn't working, I was busy with healing myself.

This was a new experience for me. I had never spent so much time on myself. Although my friend's machine did not indicate that cancer was the cause of the tumor, there was no Western medical way to know if the growth was benign or malignant without having it removed. Ultimately, I chose to have it removed. Thankfully, it was benign, and I felt relieved and grateful. The gift the whole experience has given me is a greater capacity for compassion—both for myself and others—and a deeper respect for the power of the mind-body connection.

The Story of the Perfect Heart

I love the story of "The Perfect Heart." It always reminds me that the goal in life is not to get over a loss, but to choose instead to accept what is happening with grace and love.

Once upon a time, in a time before time, long ago, there was a time when people could see inside their bodies. They could see the blood moving and the heart beating and all the organs and tissues. In the village, a young man lived who was very proud of his heart. He went around saying, "Look at me, I have a perfect heart," and people would look at his heart, which was young and strong, and say, "Yes, indeed, you do have a perfect heart."

One day, as the young man was walking around the village showing people his perfect heart, he came up to an old man sitting in a doorway.

"Look, old man, see what a perfect heart I have," he said to the old man.

The old man looked up and said, "No, you don't have a perfect heart. I have a perfect heart."

The young man looked at the old man's heart. The surface was rough and irregular; there were gouges in some places and bulges with different colors in others. "Old man," he said, "you definitely don't have a perfect heart. It's rough and irregular, not smooth like mine. And the color is all mixed up."

"Ah," said the old man, "let me explain. You see there, where a bit has a different color? That is where someone loved me so much they gave me a piece of their heart. And the colors didn't exactly match. And this place here, that is gouged out a bit? That's where I gave someone a piece of my heart but they did not give me some of theirs in return. And the places that are bumpy are where I gave a piece of my heart to someone else, and they gave me a piece of theirs in return, but it wasn't exactly the same size. So you see, this is what makes a perfect heart."

The young man looked at the old man's heart for a long time. Finally, he reached inside and took out a piece of his heart and put it in the old man's heart.

"Ah," the old man smiled, "now you're starting to have a perfect heart!"

PART TWO

A WOMAN'S LIFE STAGES AND SPECIFIC CONCERNS

Introduction

"Communities and countries and ultimately the world are only as strong as the health of their women." —Michelle Obama

Fear drives a lot of what goes on in today's medical care. Many doctors tend to project a rather pathological, fear-provoking view of women's health. They see dangers lurking behind every symptom. Doctors are not trained to recognize or be familiar with the *wide range of normal* that exists in each stage of a woman's life.

I am grateful for my years as a lay midwife that started me on my journey exploring alternatives to standard allopathic medical care for women. I am especially grateful to the opportunity it gave me to appreciate and understand the full spectrum of normal in a woman's cycles and rhythms.

Just as pregnancy has been labeled a "medical condition" with untold potential hazards, childbirth has become medicalized, and other common normal women's health variants have been pathologized (such as PMS, fibrocystic breasts, and osteopenia). Women are not reassured and told that there are wide variations within the spectrum of normal. Instead, fearful doctors encourage them to undergo unnecessary—and in some cases potentially hazardous—tests and procedures and promote controversial medications. Conventional allopathic doctors are also not trained or experienced in using the many gentle, natural, and safe methods that can be helpful to resolve women's health issues. Conventional medicine has little to offer women besides pap smears, birth control, mammograms, bone-density studies, antidepressants, and, above all, fear.

As Franklin Delano Roosevelt said, "The only thing we have to fear is fear itself." Good decisions are not made based on fear. I hope that you women reading this book find the information you need to allay your fears.

First of all, trust yourself. You alone know what is really going on in your body. No one else lives in your body and has a better observation point than you. What the tests say may or may not be helpful. The Body-Mind-Spirit is one energy, and Mind can express itself in Body, Body can express itself in Mind, and Spirit can also manifest and express in Body and/or Mind.

If you find yourself dreading your gynecological appointment... or leaving the appointment feeling that your concerns were not heard or addressed fully... or questioning whether a procedure or drug you were given is appropriate or necessary—these are signs that your alarm signal just went off. Don't brush off your intuition and emotions. Don't get herded into a hasty decision about anything. Consider finding another practitioner whom you can really partner with and who takes the time to listen to you and earns your trust. Take whatever time you need to feel certain about your choices. As an old retired doctor once advised me, "When considering options, doing nothing is an equally viable option."

Above all, trust yourself and your own knowing.

CHAPTER SIX

⌒

PUBERTY AND BEYOND

"When you're through changing, you're through."

—Martha Stewart

Puberty: Transformation from Caterpillar to Butterfly

Somewhere between the age of nine and fifteen, a girl begins her journey into womanhood. Unfortunately for humans, this metamorphosis does not occur in the safety and seclusion of a chrysalis or cocoon. Unlike butterflies, a girl's approximately seven years of pubertal transformation occur in full exposure to family and friends, as well as strangers.

The awkwardness of rapid limb growth, new hair in private places, budding breasts, and new attention from male strangers can add to a young girl's discomfort and lack of self-confidence. Madison Avenue exploits this vulnerable self-consciousness by offering a myriad of products touted to produce a smiling and self-assured presence capable of moving confidently in the public eye. Teenagers are one of the biggest markets for all kinds of products—and the advertisers know it.

Many prepubertal girls who exude confidence in their skills and capacities tell me that they do not look forward to their transformation into womanhood.

Breast Development

Remember my patient Soraya? (Her health journey is featured in the Nutrition chapter, as well as the chapter on Fatigue and Recovery). She was feeling much better at this point when I saw her—but she was worried about her eleven-year-old daughter, Sonya, whom she brought in to see me. "Sonya has this lump in her breast," Soraya explained. "My great-aunt had breast cancer, and I want you to take a look at it."

"Of course, that's a good idea," I responded, "but actually, only about 10 percent of women who get breast cancer have a family history of it." I hoped I sounded reassuring. Then, turning to Sonya, who was hovering awkwardly next to her mom's chair and looking worried, I asked her, "Is the lump painful?"

Sonya nodded.

"Which breast is it?"

Sonya put a hand to her left breast. "First this one hurt and then it stopped, and now the other one hurts. I can feel a lump there." I could see a tiny bump on her right chest through the thin T-shirt that she was wearing.

"Breast cancer is almost unheard of in young girls Sonya's age," I told her mother. "What is probably going on is an early sign of puberty." Soraya and Sonya exchanged surprised looks. With Soraya in the room, I examined Sonya's breast lump carefully and confirmed that it was, in fact, normally developing breast tissue.

I continued, "Usually, the first sign of puberty is the breasts developing little breast buds. These buds first appear as marble-sized, tender lumps beneath the areola and nipple. Often, only one breast will develop a bud at first. That one may disappear and then the other breast will develop a bud. Eventually both breasts remain larger. By the way, many boys will also develop breast buds at puberty, but they disappear as testosterone becomes dominant."

Soraya was still digesting my words. "Puberty!" she repeated. It seemed that Soraya had not anticipated her daughter entering puberty and was unprepared for its sudden appearance. Perhaps her own puberty had occurred much later, or had been accompanied by unpleasant experiences.

To relieve the tension in the air, I continued, "After breast development begins, the most common second change that happens in puberty is the growth of hair in the armpits and pubic region. Depending on one's genetic heritage, the hair may become plentiful or be rather sparse. The oil glands in the armpits also get more active and contribute to a change in strength and quality of body odor."

Sonya lifted her arm and shyly inspected her armpit. She looked relieved. "No hair yet," she reported.

I glanced at Soraya to see her reaction. Soraya looked as relieved as Sonya.

I turned to Sonya. "How do you feel about these changes? I mean, about changing from a girl to a woman?" I could see that it would be a change for her. She was muscular and lithe, and her mother had told me she spent a lot of time climbing trees and playing outside with her older brothers.

Sonya frowned and looked unhappy, "I'm not looking forward to it. Some of my girlfriends already have their periods. I don't want to stop being a kid."

It's heartbreaking to see how many young girls in our culture look at puberty with fearful anticipation and dread. I tried to sound reassuring: "Many girls feel the same as you do. And you still have a lot of years before you stop being a kid. It's important to keep being yourself and enjoying the things you enjoy doing."

Soraya asked me, "When will she start having periods?"

"You can expect menstruation to begin about a year and a half after pubic hair has developed," I answered. "A girl's puberty changes often follow the same pattern as her mother's. However, if she looks more like the women on her father's side, her puberty changes may be more similar to those of a paternal aunt or grandmother."

"I started having periods when I was thirteen," reported Soraya. "So did my sister." Sonya appeared to be listening intently to her mother's words.

Some girls begin pubertal development as young as the age of eight or nine, while others do not begin to see changes until their mid-teens. All this may be normal for a given genetic familial pattern. Some girls who are very active in gymnastics, dance, or another sport that involves strenuous workouts four and five days a week may experience a delay in the onset of the menstrual cycle. Often, the reason is that their body-fat percentage is below the level needed to support the hormones of the menstrual cycle. I have seen many girls whose menstrual cycles began only after they cut back on their participation in a super-strenuous activity.

Some girls enter pubertal development as young as the age of eight or nine, while others do not begin to see changes until their mid-teens. All this may be normal for a given genetic familial pattern.

The HPV Vaccine

"By the way," Soraya asked, "What do you think about that new vaccine for HPV? Sonya's old pediatrician was really pushing me to get her vaccinated with it."

"Yes, Gardasil or Cervarix, the vaccine for HPV, has been recommended for girls and women nine to twenty-six years old." I answered somewhat reluctantly, as this is a complicated topic.

"What is HPV?" Sonya asked.

"HPV, or Human Papilloma Virus, is a virus that lives on the surface of the skin. It is the most common STD (sexually transmitted disease) and is usually harmless and goes away by itself as the body develops immunity."

"But the ads I've seen say the vaccine will protect Sonya from getting cancer." Soraya looked puzzled.

I responded, "A few types of HPV have been linked to cervical cancer. And cervical cancer is easily detected by a pap smear—even at very early precancerous stages. What is concerning," I went on, "is that there have been numerous reports of serious adverse reactions to the HPV vaccine. The Japanese government has withdrawn the vaccine from their mandatory vaccination list. So I am not sure the benefits outweigh the risks, in this case."

Soraya looked thoughtful.

Moods

I asked Soraya, "I'm wondering if you have noticed any other changes in Sonya in the past year or so."

"Oh, yes!" Soraya nodded vigorously. "She used to be quite easygoing, but now she can be so moody!"

I nodded in commiseration. Emotional changes accompany body changes. The usually even-tempered daughter suddenly has moody spells and tantrums, or becomes more withdrawn. In the not-so-calm child, the mood changes may become more extreme and dramatic than previously. And these changes may occur in waves or can appear randomly, without warning or regularity. Emotional turbulence is another sign that the body is changing rhythms. The dance of the hormones is shifting.

> *Emotional turbulence is another sign that the body is changing rhythms. The dance of the hormones is shifting.*

Sonya had a question for me: "My cousin started having periods, but then they stopped. Is that normal?"

I assured her, "It is normal for the menstrual cycle to be irregular for the first year or longer. It may skip a month or two, then occur monthly for a few months, and then skip several or more months with no apparent pattern."

I often reassure young women that they may skip a period during times of increased stress, travel, or strenuous exercise. If periods are still very irregular or sporadic three or more years after the start of menstruation, then it is time to seek a medical evaluation to see if a medical cause can be determined.

"Since we're already on the topic of puberty," I added, "some girls notice an increase in vaginal discharge long before they start to menstruate. They may see residue in the crotch area of their underpants. This is a normal sign that their body is changing."

A Word about Vaginal Discharge

It's amazing how many women are not aware that vaginal discharge is a normal function. In my own case, it wasn't until I was in my forties that I learned that vaginal discharge is normal and healthy—not an embarrassing problem or something to be deodorized or douched away. Like our other orifices that are lined with mucous membranes, such as our nose and mouth, the vagina secretes fluids to bathe the mucous membranes and keep the area clean.

A vaginal discharge that is *not* normal will have a bad smell, or be irritating or itchy. If that occurs, one needs to see a doctor, nurse practitioner, or midwife to help figure out what may be causing the problem.

Once, many years ago, I experienced a rather foul vaginal odor and discharge, which went on for several weeks. Finally I went to the doctor—and the problem turned out to be an old tampon that had been forgotten and left inside. I was extremely embarrassed, but I was told that this kind of thing happens quite frequently. Since then, I have met several other women who had similar experiences.

If you experience a vaginal discharge—unless it has a bad smell, or is irritating or itchy (in which case, you should have a doctor check you out)—it should not be a cause for worry. It's normal!

Like our other orifices that are lined with
mucous membranes, such as our nose and mouth,
the vagina secretes fluids to bathe the mucous
membranes and keep the area clean. In most cases
a vaginal discharge is normal and should not be a
cause for worry.

GYNECOLOGICAL EXAMS

Jenn was very nervous when we first met. A trim and fit-looking woman in her fifties, she had brought along her mother and her husband for support. After we all introduced ourselves, Jenn and I went into my office, while her relatives remained in the waiting room.

Jenn was dressed in jeans and a nice shirt, without makeup, and her shoulder-length hair was brushed and pulled into a ponytail. "It's been a long time since I've been to the doctor—probably since I had kids," she revealed. "I've been pretty healthy, so far—and, well, I don't like going to doctors," she added anxiously.

"I understand," I nodded sympathetically. "Most women's experiences with doctors are pretty negative. They can be dehumanizing, and feel disrespectful too."

"Yes," she agreed, warming up a little. "I remember those awful paper gowns—I used to get so chilly waiting for the doctor in them. I've never yet met a woman who says she's looking forward to her g-y-n exam!"

I nodded my head in compassion as we both reminisced briefly about being subjected to uncomfortable pap smears and gynecological exams. I added, "I remember how humiliating it felt to meet the doctor for the first time while lying prone in those paper gowns, with my feet in the stirrups."

Jenn nodded vigorously in agreement.

"Fortunately," I went on, "in my medical school, I was trained by women who staffed the Elizabeth Blackwell Women's Clinic in downtown Philadelphia. The women would role-play as our gynecological patients, and they made sure to tell us if we were too rough, too quick, or failed to be respectful. Most medical doctors are not so lucky to get that kind of meticulous training in pelvic exams."

Jenn received this information with an expression of interest and surprise.

After reviewing what Jenn had written about her past medical history, I remarked, "You seem to be pretty healthy. It makes sense that you wouldn't need to see a doctor very often. What prompted you to make this appointment with me now?"

"Well, it's been a long time. It just felt like maybe it was time I had a checkup," Jenn replied. "Some things seem to be changing. And a friend of mine said you weren't a typical doctor, and I would probably feel more comfortable seeing you."

"How long do you think it's been since you had a pap smear?" I asked her.

Jenn looked embarrassed and said nothing.

I ventured a guess: "Twenty years?"

The expression on her face suggested that I was close.

"It really doesn't matter that much," I said reassuringly. "The guidelines for how often a woman should have a pap smear keep changing. The reason for getting pap smears is early detection of disease. But if you have been with your sexual partner for many years and are mutually monogamous, there is little chance of exposure to many of the sexually transmitted diseases."

I hoped my words were putting her embarrassment and fears to rest. "I think pap smears are over-promoted," I informed her, "and as a result many women feel guilty for not getting them more often. However, the latest guidelines suggest going every three years up to the age of thirty; then every five years; and then—for women over sixty-five, with three normal previous pap smears—none."

Concerning pap smears, the latest guidelines suggest going every three years up to the age of thirty; then every five years; and then—for women over sixty-five, with three normal previous pap smears—none.

I continued, "Routine physical exams also are over-promoted. There's no magical assurance that just because you got a physical, you won't get sick or have some major medical problem down the road. If you haven't seen a doctor in years, you probably didn't need to. You can trust that no one knows your body better than you."

Jenn looked visibly more comfortable and relaxed upon hearing this. After some more discussion, she decided to get a gynecological exam and pap smear that day. I gave her the kind of gowns I keep on hand and a sheet, and left the room so she could change.

When I returned, she was smiling. "Wow, real cloth sheets and a real cloth gown! If it had been like this years ago, I probably would have gone for exams more often."

I smiled, pleased that this respectful treatment was having such a good effect on her. But first and foremost, I wanted her to know that *she* was in control. "Before we start the exam," I told Jenn, "I want you to know that you are in charge here. If anything feels uncomfortable during the exam, please let me know. And I will tell you what I am going to do before I do it so that there are no surprises. OK?"

Jenn looked relieved. "OK," she said. And with Jenn's permission, the exam proceeded.

Anxiety is common in a woman who is about to get a gynecological exam. Many women have experienced sexual trauma, and it is important that a gynecological exam not be re-traumatizing. There have been a few times when it was clear to me that a woman was very uncomfortable, and (at her request or mine) the exam was stopped. It is very important for a woman to feel that she is in charge of her body and what happens to it. Her sense of safety overrides all other concerns.

After the exam was over and Jenn was back in her clothes, I told her, "When I get the results of the pap test, I will contact you with the results."

She thanked me and said she had a question about her daughter. "She's sixteen, now. When does *she* need to get a pap test?"

"In general," I replied, "a woman does not need to have a gynecological exam or pap test until she becomes sexually active." Jenn left the office smiling and much more at ease than when she had arrived.

> *Anxiety is common in a woman who is about to*
> *get a gynecological exam. It is very important for a*
> *woman to feel that she is in charge of her body and*
> *what happens to it. Her sense of safety overrides*
> *all other concerns.*

MENSTRUATION SUPPORT

Some of the common areas in which women may need menstruation support are cramps, heavy bleeding, and premenstrual syndrome (PMS). All these topics are covered here.

Cramps

Many women experience lower-abdominal cramping shortly before or during the first few days of their menses. There are a number of ways to reduce the pain:

- **Heat** is very effective. A heating pad or hot-water bottle on the belly can feel wonderful. You can also try adhesive heat-releasing pads that you can stick on your abdomen.
- There are **herbs,** such as raspberry leaf and cramp bark, to take as teas or as capsules.
- **Magnesium** supplements are helpful if taken during the week before your period. They help to relax the smooth muscles, including the uterus.
- **Essential oils,** such as lavender, nutmeg, cypress, and Roman chamomile work wonders. Dilute them in a little vegetable oil as a base and apply just a few drops near the nose, the soles of the feet, and on the abdomen.

- Some find that **ibuprofen** or other over-the-counter medications help relieve menstrual pain.
- It helps to get adequate and regular **sleep**.
- It also helps to eat a **healthy diet,** with plenty of fruits and vegetables.
- Some women find that after they have a baby, their premenstrual and menstrual pain is significantly less.

Heavy Menstrual Bleeding

Some women have three or four days of light menstrual flow. Others may have a day or two that is heavier, and then the bleeding tapers off. A heavy day, requiring a change in pad or tampon every three or so hours, is not a problem. Flooding, however—changing a tampon and/or a super pad every one to two hours—is problematic, and can lead to serious health concerns.

If this level of bleeding goes on for more than a day over a number of cycles, a woman can lose a significant amount of blood without realizing it. She can slowly develop an iron-deficiency anemia. A blood test to check for anemia is a good idea.

Herbs that are helpful to prevent heavy bleeding and restore balanced hormones are discussed in greater detail in the Chapter Seven: Menopause. Other tools that many women have found helpful are also in that chapter.

It is also important to avoid exogenous estrogens, such as those found in unfermented soy products, plastic water bottles, pesticide residues, and many factory-farmed animal products.

Premenstrual Syndrome (PMS)

Premenstrual syndrome, or PMS, refers to a variable period of time before a woman begins her monthly menstrual flow when she may experience a number of symptoms. The PMS period can vary in length from a few hours to up to two weeks prior to the onset of bleeding. Physical symptoms that can occur include increased breast tenderness, fluid retention, and increased gastrointestinal issues. Many women also experience increased emotional sensitivity and mood fluctuations.

Around the time of their period, women often notice being more in touch with or aware of their emotions and feelings. They may feel more vulnerable, and notice that they are quicker to get angry or burst into tears. Dr. Christiane Northrup, the well-known obstetrician-gynecologist and author of *Women's Bodies, Women's Wisdom,* tells a wonderful story about a woman who was premenstrual. She came downstairs in the morning and found her husband sitting at the kitchen table, drinking his coffee and reading the paper as usual. She burst into tears and then got mad at herself for being so emotional. Later that day, on her drive home from work, she decided to make the cornbread that her grandmother used to make. When she got home, as she began to prepare the cornbread she discovered that she was missing a key ingredient, and again she burst into tears.

What was really going on?

If we look deeper, according to Dr. Northrup, we find that the woman wanted a sign of affection and caring from her husband. She interpreted the fact that he had prepared a cup of coffee for himself but not for her to mean that he did not care about her, and burst into tears. Perhaps she herself was not aware of this yearning for more signs of caring from him. Her tears later in the day also had a deeper meaning. Grandma and her cornbread held a deep sense of home and hearth for her. She probably was not aware of her hunger to create more home-and-hearth energy in her own home, and so she could not explain why she felt so upset when she was lacking what she needed to create the cornbread.

Clues to deeper awareness: The point of this story is that we can use our PMS upsets—our angry outbursts and pronounced moods—as clues to gain deeper self-awareness. We may be ignoring important messages from our inner knowing. Or maybe we already are aware of these messages and have managed to suppress them most of the time, except during "that certain time of the month." Dr. Northrup challenges us to attend to these hints of our deeper needs and yearnings when clues arise during our premenstrual time. If we fail to do that, she warns, we are in for a rough ride when we reach menopause, as that sometimes can feel like non-stop PMS.

Premenstrual syndrome has gotten a very bad name. Perhaps we can reframe what is going on and find better ways to support women during this time in the monthly cycle. The book, *The Red Tent,* by Anita Diamont, is a fictional account of women's lives in biblical times. Before the interference of electric lights, women all menstruated at the same time in the moon cycle. Diamont describes women gathering in their own special tent—the "red tent"—when they were menstruating. There, they would spend their time making music, resting, and enjoying sisterhood and a well-needed break from their daily tasks. Even today, orthodox Jewish women sleep apart from their husbands and do not participate in sex or food preparation when they are menstruating.

The Red Tent Temple Movement, which was founded by Alisa Stark-weather, has become a popular gathering place in many cities around the world. Women host a Red Tent gathering to provide a space for other women to come, rest, relax, join a talking circle, and listen to or make music or other creative play. The activities vary, and food is usually included. It is a time for women to gather together with other women and take care of themselves. (More information on Red Tent gatherings and the website is in the Appendix, Chapter Six.)

Some women today notice that their menstrual cycle follows the moon's cycle: bleeding at the full moon, and ovulating at the time of the new moon. Many women have noticed that their cycles will synchronize with those of other menstruating women with whom they are living. One woman I know who had not menstruated for many years after a life-threatening postpartum hemorrhage began to menstruate again when her two daughters reached puberty and started their menstrual cycles.

PREGNANCY AND CHILDBIRTH

During most of my first pregnancy, my husband and I were living in Asia. Far away from my family and friends, I received very little advice or support and had access to only one book, *The New Childbirth* by Erna Wright, to prepare for childbirth. However, I felt well and had lots of energy during my pregnancy. I attended a local public prenatal clinic, and was given iron shots (which are quite painful!) for my anemia. I was young and took good health for granted, like most young folks.

In preparation for our anticipated "natural childbirth," we practiced Lamaze-style breathing, which we learned from our book. When labor started once we were back in the United States, we drove to the hospital in Topeka, Kansas, with me lying on the back seat of the car doing my Lamaze breathing. On the way, my husband got lost and I had to sit up and direct him. I was amazed that in the midst of what seemed like intense contractions, I could summon the presence of mind to make sure that we found the hospital!

I labored through the night with back labor. We had requested "natural childbirth" (a new concept, at that time) and my husband was allowed to stay with me. We were left alone for most of the night with a rare peek-in from a nurse. The doctor didn't arrive in time for the delivery. The nurses, who were trained not to keep the doctor waiting, had underestimated my progress and did not call him soon enough. It was the labor nurse who caught my baby as I pushed my daughter out. When the doctor finally arrived, he was hopping mad. His sole contribution was to jam his hand all the way into my uterus and pull out my placenta. Not a pleasant experience, and hardly part of the natural childbirth that I had planned. However, the experience of being fully awake and aware through all the sensations of labor and birth gave me increased confidence in my body and greater faith that I had the strength to be a mother.

"How Can I Best Prepare for Pregnancy and Childbirth?"

In my years as a midwife, I learned some basic precepts to enable birth to be a powerful and positive experience for mother and baby.

Precept One: It is important for a woman to give birth where she feels most safe—whether that is in a hospital, a birthing center, or at home. She will know; and it should be her choice, barring specific contraindications. Scientists have observed that if an animal is frightened while in labor, the labor will actually stop, even to the detriment of the babies. When a woman feels safe, she is best able to relax and let her body do the birthing without resistance.

Precept Two: It is very helpful to have a helper, a labor coach, or a doula at the birth whose role is to offer advice or suggestions during labor and to act as the pregnant woman's ombudsman or go-between with the physician and hospital staff. This person should be someone who is knowledgeable about the birth process, and already familiar with the laboring woman and her birth plan. This could be a friend, a relative, or a professional doula; but it should not be the woman's partner. Her partner, or primary support person, is too emotionally close to be objective. The partner's primary role is to provide emotional support for the laboring woman.

PREPARING FOR PREGNANCY AND CHILDBIRTH:

Give birth where you feel most safe.

✦

Have a helper at the birth to help you, and be a gobetween with the physician and hospital staff.

✦

There is no one "right way" to have a baby.

✦

Keep the baby with the mother after birth, if at all possible.

✦

Plan for the "fourth trimester"— the first three months after the baby's birth.

Precept Three: There is no one right way to have a baby. Each woman, and each circumstance, is unique. As a midwife, I saw many unmedicated births, as well as some births where medication and intervention—including cesarean-section delivery—were necessary and the right decision. There are many good books on pregnancy and childbirth. Being a midwife, I am partial to Ina May Gaskin's *Guide To Childbirth* (Ina May Gaskin was one of the pioneer lay midwives in the 1970s).

Precept Four: If at all possible, keep the baby with the mother once she or he is born. Request that any new-baby procedures be handled in the room with the mother. Note: if the parents don't want interventions such as prophylactic eye treatment, Hepatitis B shots, or Vitamin K shots, they need to prepare a written statement to that effect beforehand, and bring it with them to give the hospital staff.

Precept Five (MOST IMPORTANT!): Plan ahead for the "Fourth Trimester," the first three months after having the baby. It is important to get clear on who will be there to support the new mother. She will need help with shopping, cooking, cleaning, laundry, and with any young children she already has so that she can be available for the round-the-clock care that a newborn requires. Her physical, mental, and emotional wellbeing are at stake, as well as that of the whole family. If she is well supported, then the whole family benefits.

CHAPTER SEVEN

⌒

MENOPAUSE

"The wisdom that is… available to us most clearly during only certain
parts of the menstrual cycle is now potentially available all the time."
—CHRISTIANE NORTHROP, M.D., *Women's Bodies, Women's Wisdom*

HOW DOES MENOPAUSE START?

I cannot really pin down at what age I began to notice the changes associated with menopause in myself. I had a baby at age forty-four, and
was also a very busy medical resident at that time. My life was full-to-
overfull with work, baby, and family. I attributed my lack of interest in sex
to simple exhaustion; my irritability to overwork; and my night sweats to
hormonal changes from pregnancy and nursing. About the age of fifty, I
started to notice that my menstrual flow had become much lighter and
sometimes would skip a cycle. I didn't fully stop all periods until I reached
about fifty-five, but I can't quite remember (another symptom of menopause). So it's not that unusual to be uncertain what's going on as menopause begins.

THE HORMONAL CHANGES THAT TAKE PLACE IN MENOPAUSE

To understand what actually happens in women's bodies during menopause, let's review the menstrual cycle and the Dance of Estrogen and
Progesterone.

The Menstrual Cycle and Estrogen

Women secrete estrogen throughout the menstrual cycle with a surge at
ovulation. Estrogen stimulates the lining of the uterus to grow. Throughout our cycle, the lining continues to get thicker. At mid-cycle, an egg is

released from the ovary. It makes its way down through the fallopian tube into the uterus. If it is fertilized by a sperm that makes its way into the tube, the fertilized egg embeds itself within the thickened uterine lining, and begins to grow and develop into a baby. If it is not fertilized, after twenty-four hours it dies.

The Menstrual Cycle and Progesterone

At ovulation, the egg sac releases the mature egg from the ovary and begins to produce a very important hormone called progesterone. Understanding the role of progesterone is the key to understanding what is causing the changes in the menstrual cycle during the perimenopausal period.

The main function of progesterone is to stabilize and further develop the growing uterine lining, called the endometrium, to prepare for the possible implantation of the fertilized egg. The egg sac (now called the corpus luteum) is programmed to produce progesterone for about ten to fourteen days. After that, it involutes, collapses, and its work is over. If a fertilized egg has implanted, it begins to produce its own progesterone to keep the lining stable. If no egg has implanted and progesterone production from the corpus luteum has stopped, the endometrium becomes unstable and begins to fall apart and shed. Menstruation is the shedding of the thickened lining of the uterus.

Perimenopause

As women enter this seven-to-ten-year period of transition from regular cycles to none, several changes may occur. They may not produce an egg and ovulate every cycle. Even if they do ovulate, the egg sac or corpus luteum may produce less progesterone, or it may produce progesterone for fewer days.

If there is no progesterone at all or not enough to keep the uterine lining stable, the lining will reach a critical mass and begin to collapse and shed, and bleeding will result. A woman who finds that her periods have started to get closer together may be producing a decreased amount or fewer days of progesterone. If she is bleeding every two weeks or spotting and bleeding for two weeks, she may not be ovulating at all and therefore is making no progesterone to keep the endometrium from collapsing and shedding as it reaches an unstable thickness.

"I don't know what's going on with my cycles. I'm confused. Could this be menopause?" asked Jackie, a lively, vivacious blonde in her late forties. "My periods are not as regular, and sometimes I'm really moody," she added.

Over the past twenty years, I have worked with many women who have shown up at my office with change-of-life concerns. These are women who have become masterful in dancing with their monthly rhythmic dance of hormones. Now they find themselves confused. Their bodies that they have grown to know so well seem to be changing rhythms and moods. They aren't sure what's going on, but they know that something is different. There's a reason why menopause is called "The Change."

> *The bodies that women have grown to know so well seem to be changing rhythms and moods. There's a reason why menopause is called "The Change."*

"Remember when you were going through puberty?" I reminded Jackie. "Remember when your body just seemed to have a mind of its own? One day, your feet grew two sizes, and hair appeared under your arms. Your sweat smelled strong, and you needed to shower a lot more often."

Jackie nodded, a distant look in her eyes.

"Remember the awkwardness?" I went on. "And how moods would suddenly surge and overcome you, and you were in a fit of anger, or crying, and not really sure what propelled you to that state? And the agony of acne!"

Jackie laughed, "I don't know anyone who wants to go through puberty again!"

I continued, "That same feeling of being displaced—the feeling that your body has become a foreigner, an unknown entity—is what many women feel as they begin their journey through menopause. It's disorienting."

Jackie was listening intently. "It seems like my PMS goes on forever!" she remarked.

"There are many changes that happen as we head into perimenopause," I told her, nodding consolingly. "PMS symptoms that may have lasted just a day or two now may extend for one or two weeks. Many women find that their moods seem to become more pronounced."

"Yes," Jackie interjected, "I feel like a bitch half the month!"

"Welcome to perimenopause!" I responded. "Perimenopause lasts about seven to ten years from the time the hormones start to change until you have gone fourteen months without a menstrual cycle and things settle into their menopausal rhythm." I continued, "Because the rhythm of the hormones is changing, menstrual cycles start to change. They can be shorter or longer, lighter or heavier, irregular—or all of those things, in no particular order."

"Sometimes," Jackie confided, "I wake up at night, usually between 3 and 5 am, and I'm hot and covered in sweat. I have to sleep with the window open or a fan on me. Is that part of perimenopause?"

"Many women experience some degree of this. Night sweats usually happen in the week or two before the next period," I explained.

Night sweats are usually the first evidence of The Change. A woman finds herself waking at night, usually between 3 and 5 a.m., and becoming suddenly warm or hot, perhaps even breaking a sweat. This usually begins to occur in the week or two before the menses, and is the result of progesterone deficiency in the presence of adequate estrogen.

Night sweats are usually the first evidence of The Change.

Jackie nodded. "Sometimes, I can't get back to sleep for an hour or two. It's hard when you have to go to work the next morning."

I offered support: "Sleep disruption can be rough. Life starts to feel chaotic without the rhythms we have been accustomed to." Then I asked her, "Have you had any hot flashes during the day?"

Jackie shook her head. "No, thank goodness. Nothing that I've noticed, although sometimes I feel like the room is suddenly warmer—and no one else notices."

"Do certain things seem to bring on these warm flushes?" I asked her.

"Well, I have noticed that a hot shower or a glass of wine will make me feel warmer, suddenly."

Some women get waves of heat, with flushing and sweating during the day as well as at night. They find that they have to dress in layers to accommodate their inner-temperature changes.

I ventured into more personal territory. "Many women notice that their libido seems to wane, and vaginal lubrication diminishes."

Jackie looked relieved. "I really love my husband," she confided. "But I no longer feel those powerful sexual urges like I used to. My husband is understanding, but it bothers me."

If a reduced libido weren't enough of a change, there may be profound attitude shifts, as well. Many wonderful and devoted mothers start to feel that they need a break from their lives as wives or mothers, as nurturers and caregivers. Women who have been happy with their jobs or careers suddenly find them tedious and unsatisfying.

"How long is this 'change' going to go on?" Jackie wanted to know.

This is a question I have been asked a lot. "Well, just as your puberty changes took a number of years to complete, so the changes of menopause don't happen overnight. It takes about seven years, more or less, to complete the 'change' and fully enter menopause."

The changes of menopause don't happen overnight.
It takes about seven years, more or less, to complete
the "change" and fully enter menopause.

"Seven years!" Jackie looked shocked and dismayed.

I hastened to add, "On the other hand, many women are not even aware of when the 'change' began. As with puberty, some of the changes of menopause are subtle, and we may not notice them or take them as signs of the Change until hindsight makes it clearer." I pulled out a chart illustrating the flow of hormones, estrogen and progesterone, in a typical pre-menopausal cycle.

Jackie was still experiencing cycles about every four weeks. "The biggest problem is sleep interruptions from waking hot and sweaty," she complained.

Progesterone Cream

I suggested to her, "We could try using bio-identical progesterone cream, starting about day 12 of your cycle, and see if it helps with the night sweats and waking."

Jackie looked concerned. "Isn't that a hormone? I'm not sure about using hormones. Are there any side effects?"

"Bio-identical progesterone has never been shown to be dangerous or cancer promoting," I reassured her. "It is actually thought to be protective of the breast and uterus. And it promotes bone building." I added, "The most common side effect of too much progesterone is sleepiness."

"I could use that!" Jackie laughed.

Bio-identical progesterone is actually breast- and uterus-protective.

"Put the cream on at night in the 'blush zone,'" I suggested. "I mean, your upper chest and neck and face—where you blush. Some of the over-the-counter progesterone creams say to put it on your abdomen and inner thighs, but I think it works better where there is less fat under the skin and it can get into the bloodstream more easily."

Often, simply applying progesterone cream in the evening and morning will keep these night-wakings from being a problem. Many women can sail through menopause with just a little progesterone cream.

It is important to use a cream with at least 20mg of standardized pharmaceutical-grade (USP) progesterone per gram of cream. Higher-dose creams can be made by compounding pharmacies ordered by a physician. Many creams are labeled "natural progesterone." However, no natural progesterone exists outside of the body. What you want is *bio-identical* progesterone, meaning the molecule that is identical to the progesterone made by the human body. Bio-identical progesterone is synthesized from soy or wild yam. (Please note: it does not exist in the wild yam or soybean, so creams that contain only these products will not provide USP progesterone, and are not as effective.)

WOMEN'S FAMILY PATTERN OF MENOPAUSE

I had another question for Jackie: "Do you know what your mother's menopause was like? Many women's bodies follow similar development patterns to their mothers, older sisters, aunts, and grandmothers."

"I don't know much about it. She never talked about it, but I'll ask her," Jackie responded.

Genetics is important to take into consideration. It can be helpful to find out about your female relatives' menopause experiences, especially those whom you resemble in terms of other physical characteristics. This information will give you some idea of the landscape ahead. If all the women in your family ended up with hysterectomies, then they probably had problems with heavy bleeding and fibroids as they moved towards menopause. If you are aware that this might be a tendency you have inherited, you can choose to have a different story by being proactive.

HEAVY BLEEDING

"How can I stop bleeding?" My new patient, Noelle, was almost in tears. "I want to avoid a hysterectomy, if I can!" An attractive woman in her late forties, about thirty pounds overweight, she seemed frightened and worried. "I've tried birth-control pills, but they didn't work. My doctor says I should just have my uterus removed, since I don't want any more children. But I would like to keep it, if I can. Can you help me?"

Many perimenopausal women who experience long and heavy flows turn to their gynecologist for help. However, the typical gynecologist's toolbox is quite limited. Usually what is offered is either artificial hormones (which will override and suppress the body's own hormones), or a hysterectomy to get rid of that "problem" uterus. Specifically, what the gynecologists have to offer is birth-control pills, uterine ablation, uterine-artery embolization, or hysterectomy. If there are large fibroids present, then a myomectomy, or removal of just the fibroids, is another option offered. But many women who come to me are not happy with any of these choices.

In the early years of perimenopause, estrogen (unlike progesterone) continues to be produced in a woman's body. Furthermore, estrogen is made not only in the ovary but also in fat cells. Heavier women have larger amounts of estrogen, build thicker endometrial linings, and tend to bleed more heavily or longer as they move into perimenopause.

I asked Noelle, "How heavy is the bleeding? Are you bleeding through a super pad and/or tampon every hour for a day or more?"

"Yes," she replied. "Sometimes my whole bed is soaked with blood when I wake up."

I was concerned. "You are in danger of becoming anemic. We need to check your blood count."

Anemia is a sneaky phenomenon. When the blood loss through heavy menses is greater than the body's ability to replace it, then anemia is likely. However, the symptoms appear so gradually that we compensate and fail to notice. Ultimately we find ourselves exhausted, drained, and getting out of breath after climbing a flight of stairs that we used to gallop up with ease.

> *When the blood loss through heavy menses is greater than the body's ability to replace it, then anemia is likely.*

I have two friends who experienced heavy bleeding in their perimenopause years. Both chose acupuncture instead of standard gynecological treatment. Unfortunately, neither they nor their acupuncturists thought to keep a check on their blood count. After over a year of heavy monthly bleeding, one of my friends fainted in her bathroom and ended up in the emergency room, getting a transfusion and a hysterectomy. My other friend ended up nearly collapsing, and she also had a hysterectomy to end the bleeding. Both are alive and well today. I tell this cautionary tale not to warn women to avoid acupuncture for heavy bleeding—I have seen acupuncture be extremely helpful for many conditions—but to remind women, and acupuncturists, that it is important to check for anemia whenever there is heavy bleeding for more than two cycles.

I told Noelle, "I have worked with many women who would have ended up with a hysterectomy or uterine ablation, which is standard gynecological care. But together, we found gentler, safer, effective alternatives that helped ease the bleeding and allowed them to keep their uteruses intact."

"What helped them?" she wanted to know.

"There are many herbs that can help balance the hormones, reduce heavy bleeding, and provide relief from excessive hot flashes and night sweats. I use a combination of herbs in a formula called Uterine Tonic by

Herbalists & Alchemists. It includes Chaste Tree Berry, Dong Quai, Saw Palmetto, and Cyperus Root, among others."

Noelle looked interested and hopeful.

There are many herbs that can help balance the hormones, reduce heavy bleeding, and provide relief from excessive hot flashes and night sweats.

I continued, "You will need to take Uterine Tonic for at least a three-month period for it to be fully effective. It helps reduce pelvic congestion and lightens the menstrual flow, balances the hormones, and can help shrink fibroids that contribute to heavy bleeding."

Noelle was listening intently. "What do I do about the bleeding until the Uterine Tonic starts to work?"

> **HERBS THAT HELP EASE HEAVY BLEEDING:**
>
> Reckless Blood (includes Yarrow, Shepherd's Purse, Cinnamon)
>
> →
>
> Uterine Tonic (includes Chaste Tree Berry, Dong Quai, Saw Palmetto, Cyperus Root, etc.)

"I use 'Reckless Blood,' a tincture also made by Herbalists & Alchemists. It has styptic herbs such as Yarrow, Shepherd's Purse, and Cinnamon, which reduce the flooding when heavy bleeding occurs. The key with herbs is that you must use enough of them to be effective."

"How do I use it?" she inquired.

"Use a dropperful every fifteen minutes until the flow is reduced. Take more if it gets heavy again. If you have days of spotting, you can use it to stop the spotting."

"I'm excited to try the herbs!" Noelle declared. And she left the office with a bottle of Uterine Tonic and a dropper bottle of Reckless Blood.

A few days later, her blood-test results came in and I called her right away. "You are definitely anemic," I told her. "I recommend that you start taking iron supplements and eating more iron-rich foods like liver, preferably organic. Make sure the iron supplement is not ferrous sulfate, which

HELPS FOR ANEMIA:

Iron supplements (but not ferrous sulfate)

Iron-rich foods (e.g., organic liver)

can upset your stomach and cause constipation." (See the chapter on Fatigue and Recovery for more information.)

Noelle phoned me after her next period. "It was much better," she reported, "not so heavy as before." She sounded relieved and encouraged that she was on the right track for her health.

"That's great." I was happy to hear the news. "Remember to keep taking the Uterine Tonic for at least three months to get the full benefit. And use the Reckless Blood to keep the flow moderate."

Three months later, Noelle's periods were much lighter, and she was experiencing more energy than she had in a long time. She was thrilled that she had avoided a hysterectomy.

If Noelle's heavy bleeding had not resolved, I would have pursued further investigations into the underlying cause, such as:

- *A possible hormonal imbalance of estrogen and progesterone.*

- *Possible fibroids in the uterus.* Fibroids are benign fibrous growths in the uterus. Their presence can stimulate heavier bleeding.

- *A bi-manual pelvic exam.* This exam is important to get a better sense of whether the uterus or ovaries are enlarged, or whether some other abdominal condition is present. A bi-manual pelvic exam is done with one of the examiner's hands on a woman's abdomen and the other inside her vagina. This procedure allows the medical practitioner to assess the size and position of the uterus and ovaries. It is routinely done as part of a woman's gynecological exam.

- *An ultrasound of the pelvis.* This is very helpful to evaluate the uterus and ovaries, in order to determine whether there are fibroids, a thickened endometrium or uterine lining, or other abnormalities that may be contributing to heavy bleeding.

- *An underlying hypothyroid condition* that has not been detected and remedied may be the root cause for the heavy bleeding. Laboratory tests should be done that include a complete blood count, iron, and thyroid function tests. (See the chapter on Fatigue and Recovery to determine what specific thyroid and iron tests should be ordered.)

▪ Some women develop what Chinese medicine calls *dampness of the lower Chou*, or what Western medicine calls *pelvic congestion*. This condition can encourage fibroids and heavy bleeding. It can be helped with acupuncture and moxibustion, or Mayan abdominal massage therapy.

Most women sail through The Change with minor discomforts: some sleep issues, a few warm flushes during the day. However, some women suffer from severe symptoms. They have hot flashes every hour, so fierce that these women keep a fan at their desk and always dress in layers, which they tear off at regular intervals. Their faces flush and the sweat pours off. Often, they retain fluid and feel and look slightly puffy. Their rings no longer fit their fingers.

SOME HELPS FOR HOT FLASHES:

Black cohosh (herb)

✦

Remifemin

✦

Essential oils (e.g., clary sage, geranium, lemon, sage)

✦

Additional estrogen

Their symptoms usually come from a more extreme imbalance of estrogen and progesterone. I have found that making lifestyle changes, as well as using herbs and bio-identical progesterone, can reduce their menopausal lion's raging to a dull roar, or even a purr. It also helps to reduce or eliminate foods that trigger hot flashes, such as caffeine, MSG, sugar, and alcohol. Of course, it also helps to reduce the stressors in their lives.

Some women experience hot flashes, or power surges, that are frequent and severe enough to be truly bothersome and impact their quality of life. For some, black cohosh is helpful. It can be found in most health-food stores. I have often recommended the brand Remifemin, which patients have told me has helped them. Others have found relief using essential oils such as clary sage, geranium, lemon, and sage. Still others find that relief from severe hot flashes is only achieved by taking additional estrogen.

LET'S TALK ABOUT HORMONE REPLACEMENT THERAPY

Hormone replacement therapy (HRT) was developed and sold as a treatment for menopause symptoms. Prior to 2002, most doctors were quite cavalier about Hormone Replacement Therapy (HRT). They would encourage women to take Premarin at the first report of a hot flash or night sweat. If the woman still had her uterus, the doctors would prescribe Prempro, a drug that combined Premarin with synthetic progestins. Women were prescribed these hormones without the doctors ever checking the level of their patients' own hormones before starting. Nor were their hormone levels checked while the women were taking these replacement hormones. Doctors reassured women that the hormones would not only relieve them of any menopausal symptoms, but also would protect their heart, avoid osteoporosis, and keep them feeling and looking more youthful. After all, this is what the drug reps had told them.

The Women's Health Initiative Study of Hormone Replacement Therapy

All this changed in 2002, when the first results of the Women's Health Initiative study were made public. The Women's Health Initiative (WHI) was initiated by the US Government through the National Institutes of Health (NIH) in 1991. It consisted of three clinical trials and an observational study. The purpose was to address major health issues in postmenopausal women, and evaluate hormone-replacement therapy. In particular, randomized controlled trials were designed and funded that addressed cardiovascular disease, breast and colorectal cancer, and osteoporosis. The study enrolled more than 160,000 healthy postmenopausal women aged 50-79 years (at the time of enrollment) over the course of fifteen years. The study excluded women who were already diagnosed with diabetes, heart disease, or cancer.

One arm of the WHI trial gave women the drug Prempro. Prempro, made by Wyeth, consists of equine (horse) estrogens and synthetic progestins. The second arm of the trial involved women who had hysterectomies and were given only Premarin (horse estrogens), also made by Wyeth. The third was a control arm: these women took no hormones.

The study plan was to follow the women for fifteen years. The researchers expected to find that menopausal women taking estrogen and progestins (the drug Prempro) would have fewer strokes and less heart disease, osteoporosis, and breast cancer. These were claims that the pharmaceutical companies had maintained. However, the results turned out to indicate the opposite.

The study was halted after five years because the Prempro arm of the results showed a significant increase in stroke, heart disease, and breast cancer. Furthermore, there was no decrease in bone fractures. It is interesting to note that the arm of the study in which the women took only estrogen and not the synthetic progestin did not show a similar increase in breast cancer, stroke, or heart disease.

Once the WHI study was halted in 2002 and the results were revealed to doctors and the public, the use of HRT dropped significantly. Overconfidence was replaced with fear. Doctors stopped prescribing menopause hormone replacement, and women became very cautious about HRT. To this day, the WHI study continues to play a cautionary role in women's decisions regarding hormone replacement.

What mainstream medicine and the media have largely overlooked is the inappropriate methodology of prescribing hormone-replacement therapy that was used in both the WHI study and in conventional medicine. I call it the "one-size-fits-all" approach to dosing. Typically, women were given a standard dose of estrogen without first testing their individual pre-existing levels of estrogen. After they were placed on the standard dose, there was no monitoring of estrogen levels as part of the follow-up.

Mainstream medicine and the media have largely overlooked the inappropriate methodology of prescribing hormone-replacement therapy—the "one-size-fits-all" approach to dosing. The practice of giving every woman a standard dose was a major contribution to the many disagreeable and dangerous effects of hormone replacement.

This is significant. We know that not all women wear a size 9 shoe—so why should we expect that one amount of estrogen will be equally appropriate for all women? This practice of giving every woman the same standard dose was a major contributor to the many disagreeable and dangerous effects of hormone replacement. Even before the results of the WHI study became public, many women who were prescribed HRT stopped taking them soon after, because of intolerable side effects.

Bio-Identical Hormone Replacement Therapy (BHRT)

A relative newcomer in HRT is the use of bio-identical hormones in hormone-replacement therapy. Most holistic physicians as well as naturopaths are prescribing hormones that are *molecularly identical* to the ones made by the human body (hence the term "bio-identical"). Human females make only three kinds of estrogen: estradiol, estrone, and estriol. The drug Premarin, an estrogen HRT product made by Wyeth, consists of seventeen different conjugated estrogens. The name "Premarin" derives from the fact that Premarin is made from pregnant mares' urine. And, as stated earlier, human females make a specific molecule called "progesterone" that is distinctly biochemically different from the synthetic progestins found in Provera or other progestin pharmaceuticals.

Bio-Identical Progesterone Is Not the Same as Progestin

Many doctors are ignorant about the difference between bio-identical progesterone and progestins. They confuse the two and often call progestins "progesterone," unaware that they are distinctly different molecules. The drug companies have contributed to and benefitted from this confusion. To date, there is only one prescription pharmaceutical that contains bio-identical progesterone: Prometrium, a pill containing 100mg of progesterone.

Progesterone has a lot of other positive benefits besides reducing night sweats. It stimulates osteoblasts, the cells that build bone. It helps with mood and sleeplessness. It is thought to be breast-protective. Dr. John Lee, in his book, *What Your Doctor May Not Tell You About Progesterone*, details the research as well as his personal work using progesterone with hundreds of women during perimenopause and menopause. In my own experiences with bio-identical progesterone I found it to be helpful, with a few exceptions.

Bio-identical Hormone Replacement Therapy (BHRT) uses various combinations of estradiol, estrone, estriol, progesterone, and testosterone. These hormones are pharmaceutical-grade and synthesized in approved laboratories. They are identical in molecular structure to hormones made in the human body. They may be given in combination or taken individually. Sometimes other bio-identical hormones such as testosterone and DHEA are added.

The holistic physician or naturopath who prescribes BHRT must first evaluate a woman's current level of hormones, and then—based on her symptoms and her existing levels of hormones—prescribe a combination of hormones to be taken, either as a pill, cream, drops, or sublingual lozenges. Once the woman is taking the hormone replacement, her levels of hormones should be carefully monitored at regular intervals to ensure that they stay within the physiological normal range. Some doctors have prescribed bio-identical hormones in the form of a pellet that is injected under the skin. I personally have not used this method, as I find it too difficult to regulate.

Pharmacists who specialize in compounding are able to prepare these unique and personalized combinations and dosages of bio-identical hormones. These compounding pharmacies used to be quite rare. One of the first that I learned about was the Women's International Pharmacy in Madison, Wisconsin. They still offer the same user-friendly service and helpful information as they did when I first began to work with them. These days, compounding pharmacies are popping up everywhere. Pharmacists who want to do more than just pill counting are excited at the prospect of customizing products for individual needs. Many also make all manner of creams for pain as well as other special products. These compounding pharmacies also are a good resource for finding doctors in your area who prescribe bio-identical hormones.

Some women have asked me if I would prescribe the so-called Wiley Protocol, which is described in Suzanne Somers' book, *The Sexy Years*. Suzanne touts the use of bio-identical hormones in a complicated dosing pattern that returned her to a monthly bleeding cycle after menopause. I am personally leery of using a level of hormones that is high enough to cause the endometrial lining to build to a point that results in monthly bleeding.

I have not heard of any increased incidence of breast cancer, stroke, or heart disease in women using bio-identical hormones in monitored physiological doses. Bio-identical hormone therapy has been available in Europe for decades now, and no reports have emerged showing that they put women at greater health risk. If you are having significant menopause symptoms and have found little or no relief working with herbs, acupuncture, and dietary interventions, I would suggest that you give bio-identical hormones a try. It is important to check hormone levels at least once a year if you are taking supplemental hormones.

If you are having significant menopause symptoms and have found little or no relief working with herbs, acupuncture, and dietary interventions, I would suggest that you give bio–identical hormones a try.

OSTEOPOROSIS

Osteoporosis has become a big concern for women since the onset of bone-density testing. Many women over fifty are chided regularly by their gynecologist to get a bone-density study. Somehow, men are not expected to get bone-density testing, although men can also lose bone as they age. Most people, according to the bone-density studies, lose some bone density as they age.

The big concern at the bottom of all this fuss about bone density is hip fractures. It is well known that most elderly people who suffer a hip fracture usually die about a year and a half later, and that their health is likely to be seriously compromised as a result of the fracture. What follows are frequently asked questions (FAQs) that I hear about osteoporosis.

"Should I Get a Bone-Density Study?"

The basic question to answer, whenever you are considering any test or medical procedure is: "Will the results of this test affect my choice of treatment?" If you would not do anything differently, regardless of the results of a particular test or procedure, then reconsider whether it is important to do the test. Sometimes, people choose to do a test in order to evaluate how a treatment course is going or to get a baseline value. It is also important to balance the benefit of the additional information that the test or procedure may provide with the risks that the test or procedure may incur. Risks in a bone-density study include radiation exposure as well as erroneous interpretation of results, which may generate undue fear.

"What Does a Bone-Density Study Measure?"

A bone-density study is basically an extensive series of X-rays to measure the thickness of our bones. Certain bones—the neck of the femur and the lumbar spine vertebrae, in particular—have been chosen to be studied, and the thickness measurements are compared to those of twenty-five-year-old women.

The issue I have with the bone-density study is this: it is an evaluation of the *thickness* of the bone, not the *resilience* of the bone. Just because a bone is thick does not mean that it has the kind of tensile strength needed to withstand trauma such as a jarring blow, an abrupt bend or twist, and torsion. What we need are *strong, flexible bones*, not necessarily thick bones. To date, there is no good evidence that just because a bone is thicker, it has more tensile strength. Likewise, the evidence is not clear that thinner bones are less flexible or have less tensile strength.

> *What we need are strong, flexible bones. Just because a bone is thick does not mean that it has the kind of tensile strength needed to withstand trauma such as a jarring blow, an abrupt bend or twist, and torsion.*

"What Is Osteopenia?"

If the bone-density study reveals some bone loss, it is then graded as either "osteoporosis" or "osteopenia." Osteopenia is a term that was created by the bone-density-study developers to denote the presence of bone loss that is less than what is technically defined as osteoporosis. However, for all we know, osteopenia may be the *normal condition* of bone in older people. We don't actually know very much, because bone-density studies haven't been around very long.

Nevertheless, being given the diagnosis of osteopenia sounds quite worrisome and a little scary. Many women have come to me frightened about their diagnosis. They ask me whether they should take the drugs the physicians recommend.

The primary drugs used to thicken bone are a class called bisphosphonates. To date, there is no clear evidence that a bone that has been made thicker through the use of bisphosphonates actually has a reduced risk of fracture. Furthermore, the way these drugs work is by disrupting osteoclast activity. The result is that the old, broken microcrystals of bone are no longer removed before being paved over by new bone. Naturally, the bone will appear thicker—but is it stronger? Perhaps it is just thicker and more brittle. Bisphosphonates—besides having dubious positive effects—also have several very worrisome potential side effects. One is that they can cause erosion of the esophagus, if swallowed incorrectly; and another is the potential for total necrosis of the jawbone, which is irreversible. Good to note: the FDA has issued a warning about this class of drugs.

My experience with patients who have bone-density studies is that these studies provoke anxiety and fear. They also involve a lot of radiation exposure and promote the use of unhelpful and potentially harmful drugs. I don't recommend them. Instead, I suggest that women use the four strategies (under the heading "How Do I Build and Maintain Strong Bones?"—see below) that are known to help maintain healthy strong bones.

How Bones Work

It is important to understand that bone—like skin, nerves, and muscle—is living tissue. Bone has a thin periosteal membrane coating it, providing connection to the nervous system. It has blood vessels running through it that bring nutrients and carry away waste material. Bone tissue is in the form of three-dimensional microcrystals. These crystals sometimes break as a result of normal wear-and-tear on the body. Shin splints are an example of more extensive microcrystalline fractures in the shin area that can occur due to repetitive stresses such as running.

To repair these microcrystalline fractures, bone is constantly undergoing remodeling. Osteoclasts and osteoblasts, two types of bone cells, are the remodelers. The osteoclasts break down old broken or fractured crystals, and the osteoblasts form new bone. It reminds me of the sidewalks in the neighborhood where I grew up. As the trees near the sidewalk grew bigger, their roots often cracked the sidewalk. A crew of city maintenance men would come through and dig up the old fractured sidewalk, and then another paving crew would come through later and lay down the new sidewalk. It was an ongoing process of removing and replacing—similar to bone maintenance..

"How Do I Build and Maintain Strong Bones?"

Bone has four requirements to remain vital and strong.

1. A good diet rich in bone nutrients.
2. Adequate levels of Vitamin D3, in order to absorb the calcium and other minerals.
3. Our digestion must be in good order to enable us to absorb the minerals in our diet.
4. Our bones need to be stimulated with activity to stay strong.

1. A good diet rich in minerals and bone nutrients.

A good diet contains lots of the nutrients that bones need. Contrary to popular belief, bones need *all* the minerals, not just calcium, in order to be strong. Furthermore, a lot of cheaper bone-building supplements out there contain calcium carbonate, which is made from limestone and oyster shells. I don't know about you, but I cannot digest oyster shells—or limestone, for that matter. I don't recommend the carbonate form of calcium. Better, more absorbable, forms of calcium are calcium citrate, glycinate, ascorbate, and gluconate.

A diet that is varied—with lots of leafy green vegetables, a variety of animal meats and fish, nuts, and whole-grains—will contain the many macro- and micro-nutrients that bone needs. Bone broth is another really good source of minerals. (See Appendix B for instructions on how to make bone broth.)

2. Adequate levels of Vitamin D and sunshine.

Adequate levels of Vitamin D are essential for absorption of calcium. The blood test that you want to order specifically checks Vitamin D3, 25, and OH. I have checked many people's Vitamin D levels over the years, and

I am shocked at how many men, women, and children have low levels, or are at the low end of the normal range.

Yes, it's true: our bodies can synthesize Vitamin D3 when we expose ourselves to sunshine. However, it seems that these days, even children are not outside long enough, with enough skin exposed, to produce adequate amounts. In addition, sun exposure is less effective in the winter, when the sun's angle to the earth is more acute and sunlight is less intense. The intensity of the sunlight also decreases the closer you live to the poles.

For years, we have been taught that the use of sunscreen is a good thing to prevent later development of skin cancer. Sunscreen decreases the UVB exposure. However, UVB is *needed* for the critical conversion of Vitamin D2 to D3, the active form of the vitamin. In reality, what causes skin cancer is repeated severe sunburn, not just sun exposure. Most of the people who develop skin cancers had lots of bad, blistering sunburns in their past. Remember: skin cancer is not deadly, just unpleasant. Maybe skin cancer should be renamed skin dysplasia, as it doesn't act like other cancers that spread within the body to other organs. Skin cancer like squamous or basal-cell carcinoma stays on the surface of the skin. Melanoma, however, is a very different kind of skin cancer, which starts in the skin and can later become metastatic throughout the body and deadly. Melanoma is not caused by sun exposure, and often appears on parts of the body that are rarely exposed to the sun.

To conclude, some exposure to direct sunshine is a good thing. It seems that our fears of sun exposure were overblown (though it did sell a lot of sunscreen lotion). The key to adequate sun exposure is moderation: don't overdo it, and don't get burned.

Most people need to take supplemental Vitamin D3 (cholecalciferol) to get their levels in a good range. I generally recommend taking 5,000 IU daily to maintain Vitamin D in the range of 50-60, in labs that have a 30-100 range. If your levels are below the normal range, you may need to take 10,000 IU daily for a month and then drop back to a maintenance dose of 2,000-5,000 IU per day. Some exposure to direct sunshine is a good thing.

Many doctors prescribe Vitamin D2, which comes in a 50,000 IU dose and requires a doctor's prescription to obtain. Unfortunately, without adequate sun exposure, this will not be converted to the active D3 form. It is also important to take supplemental Vitamin D3 with a meal, because it is fat-soluble and you want the digestive enzymes to be activated in order to maximize its absorption.

3. A well-functioning digestion that can absorb minerals.

Our digestion must be in good order to enable us to absorb the minerals in our diet. If you are having trouble with heartburn, reflux, gas, diarrhea, or constipation, it means that your digestion is not working optimally.

Time for a tune up! Review the material in the Chapter Two, "Engaging the Rhythms of Good Digestion," to evaluate what you need in order to have a good digestive function. If your digestion is not working well, you are wasting all the precious minerals and other nutrients in your food and supplements. You might as well just throw them directly down the toilet.

4. The need to move and use our bodies.

Our bones need to be stimulated with activity to stay strong. Weight-bearing activity is very important. When we move, our muscles contract, and the tendons and ligaments that attach them to bone pull on the bone, creating stress and strain. That stress is necessary to stimulate bone growth.

It is not that hard to find weight-bearing activities. They look like taking out the trash, raking the leaves, vacuuming or sweeping, carrying the groceries, walking, swimming, dancing. or bicycling, to mention a few. At least 30 minutes a day is good. Some people find using a pedometer or one of the fancier tracking devices helpful to stay aware of how active they actually are.

Extra Tidbits about Developing Strong Bones

There are two homeopathic remedies that seem to promote bone development. One is called Calc phos, or Calcarea phosphoricum. For this purpose, the 6X or 6C strength is best—a few pellets once a day, melted in the mouth, then avoid food for fifteen minutes after taking them.

The other remedy is called by various names—Bioplasma or Twelve Tissue Salts, depending on which homeopathic company has manufactured it—and is a combination of twelve different mineral salts in homeopathic dosage. Take approximately 1/8 teaspoon of pellets once daily, melted in the mouth. As with all homeopathics, wait fifteen minutes after taking them before eating. (There is more information on homeopathy in the Appendix.)

My mother was a tiny woman with very small bones and a pronounced kyphotic spine. In her later years, she certainly fit the stereotypical picture of the osteoporotic elderly woman. (She also smoked a pack of Camels a day and ultimately died of emphysema complications—but that's another story.) Although she never took vitamins or any supplements, I had persuaded her to take a few homeopathic pellets of Calc phos 6X, which she did every morning. I think she liked them because they tasted sweet.

One day when she was well in her eighties, she fell over some big boxes in her hall and developed a huge bruise that went from her pelvis all the way down her thigh to her knee. If her tiny, thin bones had been weak or brittle, they would definitely have been broken in that fall. Instead, she just had bruises. Her doctors were surprised. I think the

BUILDING STRONG BONES:

To get enough Calcium—in the form of calcium citrate, glycinate, ascorbate, or gluconate:

A varied diet, including:
Leafy green veggies
Various animal meats
Fish
Nuts
Whole grains
Bone broth

To get enough Vitamin D:

Ensure moderate exposure to the sun

Take Vitamin D3 (2-5000 IU daily with a meal)

Regular weight-bearing exercise

Homeopathic remedies that promote good bones:

Calcarea phosphoricum (6X or 6C)

Bioplasma (aka "Twelve Tissue Salts")

Calc phos might have made a difference. Of course, it could also be that she had strong bones from good nutrition through her life or genetics, or just plain good luck with the fall.

Another bone-building promoter is the hormone progesterone. Progesterone stimulates the osteoblasts, the bone cells that make new bone. I have had patients show improvement in bone density on their bone-density studies after using progesterone cream in addition to the "four things that build Bone." How much progesterone? About a pea-size dab, twice daily, of a cream that contains 20 mg of progesterone per gram of cream. Using more is not life-threatening. The most common secondary effect of progesterone is sleepiness. (This actually may be a benefit, if sleep problems are an issue.) Some women use it only at night, or use less in the morning. The best places to put the cream are areas with minimal fat below the skin, such as the upper chest, neck and face, inner elbows, and behind the knees.

POST-MENOPAUSAL ZEST

Margaret Mead, the famous anthropologist, spoke of a "post-menopausal zest." I have seen women in their fifties, sixties, seventies, and beyond who have this zesty, feisty spirit. This is the woman who is not afraid to dress for her own enjoyment, who speaks her mind and stands in her truth. The woman who finds life a continuing unfolding adventure—who is open to new ideas and experiences—is living a zesty life.

Older women have not been given much recognition in our culture. They have become synonymous with "useless," "dried-up," and invisible. We rarely see them on television or in the movies. Their wrinkled faces don't smile at us from magazine ads and billboards.

Strangely, despite the cultural bias, many women find a new kind of strength as they age. They no longer wait to be asked for their opinion. They have grown comfortable speaking up and telling their truth, regardless of the consequences. They can be quite firm and unyielding in their position on politics, social issues, and whatever other causes they choose to champion. Many profound social changes are the result of older women who spent their lives dedicated to creating a better world for children, women, families, the poor, and the environment.

Here is a short list of older women who became great role models in their later years:

Aung San Suu Kyi, Alice Walker, Billie Jean King, Maya Angelou, Angela Merkel, Sonia Soto-Meyer, Georgia O'Keeffe, Rachel Carson, Germaine Greer, Gloria Steinem, Marie Curie, Elizabeth Blackwell, Margaret Mead, Simone De Beauvoir, Wangari Maathai, Madonna, Judy Chicago, Joan Baez, Angela Davis, Pema Chodron, Oprah Winfrey, Jane Goodall, Eleanor Roosevelt, Candace Pert, Vandana Shiva, Margaret Sanger, Grandma Moses, Tillie Olsen, Harriet Tubman, Hildegaard von Bingen, Susan B. Anthony, Mother Teresa, Coco Chanel, Dorothy Day, Rita Moreno, Ruth Bader Ginsberg, Vivian Westwood, Ninette Devaloir, Martha Graham, Helen Keller, Marion Woodman, Niki de Saint Phalle, and Tony Morrison.

These older women found their port-menopausal zest. Once done with childbearing and rearing, they took their creative energy out into the world. They followed their vision with a lot of hard work and dedication. Reading some of their biographies and autobiographies is inspiring. Some of them managed great achievements against huge obstacles.

CHAPTER EIGHT

SEXUALITY

"Sex is a foretaste of the world to come." —Talmud Brachot 57-B

Our Sex Drive: What Is a Healthy Sexual Appetite?

Once we reach the age of reproduction, our sex drive is joined with Life's own drive to continue Life. In nature, plants develop flowers to entice their pollinators in order to produce the seeds of the next generation. Animals and insects create pheromones that attract a mate. Although many young people are unaware of an urge to procreate, they are drawn to sexual activity after puberty. For some, this sexual drive can be extremely strong, while others have never had a huge sexual appetite.

When teenagers are no longer small enough to fit on mommy's or daddy's lap, many of them still hunger for connection and physical touch. That hunger may be diverted into sexual contact. In many other parts of the world, it is common to see young men and women walking together hand-in-hand or arm-in-arm with friends of the same sex. In the US, homophobia has inhibited this natural tendency to touch and physically connect with those close to us. At the same time, we are barraged with images of sexual love in the media. Many teenagers today turn to sex as a means of satisfying their need for touch, sensuality, love, and connection.

Gender

In Thailand, I have been told, twenty-one different genders are recognized. We in the US are exploring gender expression and how to language it appropriately. There is the gender you were born with, which may have been ambiguous. There is the gender you identify yourself as being. There is the gender that you are attracted to sexually. And there are many variants in each of these categories.

TRAUMA

If we have experienced sexual trauma or abuse in our childhood, this can deeply affect our sexuality, whether we are conscious of it or not. Traumatic experiences are stored in our bodies—in the collagen in the tissues—as well as in our conscious and unconscious memories. The trauma can be retriggered by touch, as well as by smell, taste, or any other of our five senses. (A more complete explanation of the process of PTSD—Post Traumatic Stress Disorder—can be found in Chapter Five: "Emotion: The Mind-Body Connection.")

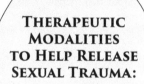

THERAPEUTIC MODALITIES TO HELP RELEASE SEXUAL TRAUMA:

Acupuncture

✢

Reiki

✢

Somatic Experiencing

✢

Gestalt therapy

✢

Shamanic work

✢

EMDR

✢

Talk therapy

"My sexuality seems blocked—what can I do?" Anya almost whispered these words to me at our first appointment as she sat tensely in her chair. Her tone and body language conveyed the depths of shame and misery she was experiencing.

Anya shared with me that she had been sexually abused as a young child. For many years, those early traumatic sexual experiences had been forgotten and stored below her consciousness. She had enjoyed sexual activity during her teen years and into her twenties. However, after she reached her thirties, the memories began to re-emerge. She became aware of a deep anger and felt numb and discomfort with sexual touch.

"Many victims of childhood abuse experience what you are going through," I reassured her. "It's a terrible thing, and I'm so sorry it happened to you. What's encouraging is that now that you are conscious of these feelings and memories, you can begin the process of healing from these old wounds."

Together, Anya and I reviewed some of the many therapeutic approaches that are available to help with her healing journey.

Many therapeutic approaches are available to help with the journey to heal from sexual trauma.

Many amazing healing modalities are available to work through these blocks and release the trauma from the body. I have seen people helped by acupuncture, Reiki, Somatic Experiencing, gestalt therapy, shamanic work, shadow work, talking with a therapist, and a number of other modalities. Some of the modalities mentioned in Chapter Five: "Emotion: The Mind-Body Connection" can also help, such as EMDR and Rapid Resolution Therapy.

BODY IMAGE

As women, we have been given strong messages that have affected our attitude towards our bodies and our sexuality. Sometimes we don't feel sexual because we don't feel good about our bodies.

Lots of women become unhappy when they look in the mirror. We can thank the media for the promotion of a thin, firm-breasted, long-legged twenty-something-year-old as the image of beauty. Few women look like this young ideal, even in their twenties. What's more, the farther you travel from twenty, the more likely that you won't look like the twenty-year-old in the ads.

The media isn't stupid. The obvious implication that women should look a certain way promotes sales of makeup, Spanx, tanning creams, teeth-bleaching kits, push-up bras, and much more. The strategy has worked well for them. But it's not working so well for women in terms of their self-image and their sexuality.

What can women do to restore their confidence in their own intrinsic beauty and value as women? Personally, I find it refreshing to watch old Mae West movies. Mae was by no means a beauty by our modern standards. Yet with every movement, gesture, and word she spoke, she revealed her awareness that she was a confident, sensual, powerful, intelligent, unique, and fully embodied woman. What's more, to my surprise, the credits revealed that Mae had also written the screenplays! I started practicing my "Mae West walk" on my morning ambles and found that it created a newfound self-confidence and pride in my womanhood.

The recent loosening of rigid sexual identities has created more breathing room for individuals to explore their own unique sexuality. With the relaxation of gender identity, new concepts of beauty are evolving. There are many ways a woman can heal a negative self-image that is impacting her, and discover her own intrinsic beauty and unique value.

IS IT SEX OR IS IT LOVE?

Many people equate or conflate love with sex, and sex with touch. They use sex to fulfill their needs for touch, or they confuse sexual pleasure with love. I can understand how this can happen. I have experienced this myself, and have mistakenly thought that because someone gave me sexual pleasure, they loved me. Perhaps many of us have traded sex for love or love for sex at some time in our life.

And the converse is also true: it is a mistake to assume that someone doesn't love you because they are not interested in being sexual with you. In our society, sex and love are often confused or conflated. Do we need to have sex to feel loved? I have met many people who have told me that they feel loved and physically satisfied in their relationship with their partner even though they no longer are sexually active. They still enjoy physical affection in the form of hugs and cuddling with their partners. I have also met others who are partnered and sexually active but do not feel satisfied with their sexual life. Sexual dissatisfaction or satisfaction can occur both with those who are having sex and those who are not.

Sexual satisfaction is important. However, what that means for each individual is entirely unique to them—and also unique for that moment in their life. And, like everything else in life, our sexual and sensual needs change. What satisfied us as a child changes when we become a teenager, and is different again in our twenties, our thirties, our forties, fifties, sixties, and on. As we grow older, our sexual drive naturally undergoes changes.

Sexual satisfaction is important. However, what that means for each individual is entirely unique to them—and also unique for that moment in their life.

KNOW YOURSELF

One key to sexual and sensual satisfaction is to know what pleases you. It is helpful to spend time discovering your own body and what is pleasurable... what feels good... what delights and what does not.

A very informative book is Betty Dodson's *Sex for One*. Betty Dodson spent many years traveling and teaching workshops on the art of self-pleasuring to both men and women. Her book provides many insights into the amazing and unique ways that we are all different, as well as reassurance and encouragement in our journey of discovering our sensual and sexual joys.

Masturbation can provide sexual satisfaction for women who are not partnered for reasons of choice or circumstance, and it can also add to the sexual repertoire of couples. According to Betty Dodson, "Masturbation is a primary form of sexual expression... Masturbation is a way for all of us to learn about sexual response. It's an opportunity for us to explore our bodies and minds for all those sexual secrets we've been taught to hide, even from ourselves. What better way to learn about pleasure and being sexually creative? We don't have to perform or meet anyone else's standards, to satisfy the needs of a partner, or to fear criticism or rejection for failure. Sexual skills are like any other skills; they're not magically inherited, they have to be learned."

Another wonderful book that can help guide you in your journey of sexual/sensual education is *Women's Anatomy of Arousal: Secret Maps to Buried Treasure*, by Sheri Winston. Her book even includes highlighted sections entitled "Hot Tips for Guys."

In her research, Sheri Winston discovered that the description of the physiology of the clitoris underwent a revision during the Victorian era. Prior to then, it was understood that a woman's sensitive and erectile tissue included not only the clitoris but extended into the labia, the floor of the perineum, and the vagina. The Victorians re-defined a woman's erectile tissue to include only the small appendage below its tiny hood at the junction of the labia. So the Victorians changed the physiology text-books—and the texts haven't been revised since. Even today, doctors as well as many others continue to be misinformed.

However, thanks to Sheri Winston's research, we can reclaim what we may have intuitively felt or discovered for ourselves but had no scientific data to support: in fact, women have as much sensitive erectile tissue as men. When a woman is fully sexually aroused, this erectile tissue swells with extra blood in the same manner as a man's erectile tissue.

Naomi Wolf's book, *Vagina*, reveals a little-known fact that each woman's genital area is unique in its neurological arrangement, unlike men who are basically all wired the same. In *Vagina*, she describes her fascinating journey to understanding female sexuality.

With regard to heterosexual relationships, I have found two books by Alison Armstrong, *Keys to the Kingdom* and *The Queen's Code*, to be very helpful in clarifying both male and female perspectives on love and sex. She has many good suggestions to improve good communication between men and women.

And at the core—and perhaps our greatest challenge—is self-love: to value and honor our own existence as worthy and good. Self-love honors our own needs, and has compassion for our imperfections and frailties. We are, after all, only human.

> *Self-love is at the core: to value and honor our own existence as worthy and good. Self-love honors our own needs, and has compassion for our imperfections and frailties.*

SEX AFTER MENOPAUSE

Remember my menopausal patient, Jackie, from Chapter Seven: "Meno-pause"? She returned after using bio-identical progesterone cream for a period of time. "I am definitely sleeping better when I remember to put on the cream," she reported. "But I have another question: What happened to my sex drive? I'm just not that interested in sex, these days."

Our sex drive goes through some changes with the onset of the per-imenopausal period—changes just as dramatic as those we went through in puberty. Some women (like some men) never had a very big sex drive in the first place, in which case the changes in their sex drive caused by menopause may not be a source of difficulty for them. But for those women who previously enjoyed a robust sex drive, it is confounding and disturbing to them to observe their sex drive falter and fade. These women also worry that their sexual partners may be dissatisfied with their change in sexual responsiveness.

We have biology to thank for some of this. Biology uses the sex drive to make babies. Many menstruating women have noticed that their desire for sexual intercourse greatly increases right around the time when they ovulate and are most likely to get pregnant. When ovulation ceases at menopause, that biological drive to make a baby also goes away.

However, what does *not* go away is the desire and the need for physical touch, for pleasure, and for intimacy. As human beings, we will always enjoy and need touch, no matter our age. I often suggest to my patients that they let go of their old expectations and focus on discovering their new sexual and sensual menopausal selves. Many older women notice that it takes more time to become sexually aroused and orgasms may be less frequent.

In *Vagina*, Naomi Wolf quotes Caroline Muir, a tantra teacher, speaking about older women's orgasms. Muir said, "There are waves of orgasmic energy. When you are twenty, you have hot, fast orgasms. When you are older, they soften and get more intense. The pathways between genitals and brain have had more years to wake up. There are more pathways, so it feels different from fast, hot clitoral orgasms."

It can be helpful to spend time re-learning what and how to touch in order to get sexually aroused. Sheri Winston's *Women's Anatomy of Arousal* and Betty Dodson's *Sex for One* are very helpful resources for good information about women's sexual-arousal possibilities, whether the woman is single or partnered.

Vaginal dryness can make intercourse uncomfortable and less enjoyable. A number of companies sell sexual lubricants, and some of my patients find coconut oil a good option. The herbal tincture, Replenish, made by Herbalists and Alchemists, is wonderful for restoring moistness to vaginal tissue as well as eyes and mouth. The aphrodisiacal effects of cannabis have been well documented, used both topically and as an oral supplement or smoked.

Bio-identical hormones can be helpful for some women when pain with intercourse prevents them from continuing to be sexually active. Some women find that adding bio-identical testosterone helps improve their libido. (More information on hormone replacement therapy is in Chapter Seven: "Menopause.")

If you are partnered, it helps to have open and honest communication with your partner. Older men have their own issues with sexual drive and performance. To their merit, many older men become less focused on their own sexual release and are more interested in pleasing their partner than when they were young. There are many variables that influence sexual drive and how a couple adjusts to menopause.

An older-man friend of mine described his experience with what he calls "the great gift of mature physical love":

> *"Now I'm a grandfather having sex with a grandmother, and the mainstream culture finds that a very unattractive situation. With endless images of athletic young people (or the occasional middle-aged one who still looks like a young person) being the only acceptable ideals for a gratifying sex life, what are we going to do? These images also burden men, as they have been conditioned to an unrealistic image of beauty.*
>
> *"I'm going to tell you a secret some of us hip oldsters have been hiding from you foolish naïve youngsters: You can go to bed with a wrinkled grandmother and when she gets turned on, everything changes, all the good stuff gets engorged. Her pussy gets engorged. The labia and clitoral bulbs swell up. The urethral sponge swells up. It gets real snug and juicy in there.*
>
> *"It doesn't stop down there. Her face engorges and becomes smooth, her wrinkles are gone, and her skin literally glows. The grandmother you went to bed with is now a radiant Love Goddess.*
>
> *"You could say she looks young, and that's true in a way; but it doesn't do justice to what she's become. 'Young' can be firm and pretty, but not deep and rich with mature wisdom and sexual talent. like this one. And I don't look anything like the man she was gazing at across the dinner table either. It works both ways.*

"And this is only the beginning. Our boundaries are more open. Our sensitivities to each other are more enhanced. Our capacity to feel our own pleasure and our partner's enters into a circular gestalt, where we feel more than ever before the actual pleasure our partner is feeling from what we are giving them. We actually become positive, multidimensional feedback loops as existing forms of pleasure morph through an apparent endless play of new wonderful experiences, bringing awe and humor and the promise of so much more in this open-ended love play.

"This is the great gift of mature physical love between people who have developed an open and honest relationship."

REMEMBER APHRODITE!

Aphrodite is the goddess of Love and Sensuality. She cultivates Beauty. Hers is the garden of pleasures and delights. Once the busyness of raising children or career demands lessens, women find they have more time to cultivate their inner Aphrodite. We can take the time to explore what brings us pleasure and joy.

Some women find they have an increased interest in sexual play after menopause, when the fear of unwanted pregnancy is no longer a factor. Whether partnered or alone, a woman can find ways to feel sensually and sexually pleasured at any age.

There is joy to be found in the sensual as well as sexual nature of life—the push and pull you feel standing in the ocean surf, the delight of a shower, the sun's warming touch, the softness of a feather, the rich taste of chocolate, the pleasure of a massage. Activities such as eating, dancing, walking, swimming, and many more have rich sensual delights to offer. Sometimes a glass of wine or a few puffs of marijuana can enhance the sensuality of the moment.

According to Jean Shinoda Bolen, M.D., in *Goddesses in Older Women*: "Later-life passions may turn out to be more unconventional as well as highly personal choices. Aphrodite can imbue a relationship between two people with love and beauty; and unadulterated joy can result especially in two older people, who know how blessed they are to have found each other at this stage of life and whose friends and relatives are delighted for them."

Sexuality and sensuality are our birthright as we embody the archetype Aphrodite. We were created to enjoy being alive in this world. To feel caressed by a breeze, serenaded by the birds' songs, taste a mango, move our body—these are some of the sensual joys that can be ours. Nourishing our need for sensual pleasure in all the myriad possible manifestations is a practice that we can continue to cultivate throughout our lives.

CHAPTER NINE

~

FATIGUE AND RECOVERY

"Hopefully one day, my dream is that our medical community will produce a formal apology to the patients that—not having believed them all these years—they are facing a real illness."

—DR. JOSE MONTOYA, CFS researcher and clinician, Stanford University (during a lecture on Chronic Fatigue Syndrome at Stanford University, March 3, 2011)

"I am sick and tired of feeling tired all the time!" Fatigue is one of the most common issues that bring people to my practice. Fatigue can result from many different conditions, including physical, mental, and emotional.

We were not taught about Chronic Fatigue Syndrome in medical school. Instead, we were told that patients who continued to complain about lack of energy and whose blood tests were normal were "malingerers": that some people were "chronic whiners" or just wanted to stay sick for some ulterior motive, or maybe they were "depressed." Unfortunately, many doctors continue to have this mindset today. Even those doctors who *do* believe their patients use the diagnosis of "Chronic Fatigue Syndrome" (CFS) as basically a waste-basket term to mean, "We believe you are really tired, and we don't know the reason why."

CHRONIC FATIGUE IS NOT SOMETHING MADE UP BY "MALIN-GERERS"

While there may be a small subset of people who might fit the label of "malngerers," I don't think I have met one yet. I have met many people in my own practice for whom long-standing fatigue is a *real* problem, and they are *desperately* trying to find a solution. They don't want to stay tired. They want to get back to living a full life. They have been to doctor after doctor, had numerous lab tests, and tried antidepressants, stimulants, and numerous other prescription drugs—all with little success in resolving their underlying fatigue. The 15-minute office appointment practiced in medicine today allows little time to delve into the history of a patient's chronic fatigue. Standard conventional medical care offers such patients little chance of achieving a real resolution for their chronic fatigue. They want to dance with the Rhythms of life, but they have been sidelined by their fatigue—doomed to be wallflowers at the dance.

Thomas is a good example. An air-traffic controller for over twenty years, he was 51 when he first came to me for health advice. "I don't have the energy I used to have," he complained. "I'm not sleeping well, and my job is very stressful. Plus, it doesn't help that my work schedule is different every day." Despite his loss of energy, he had managed to keep up a very busy life, including participating in many weekend bicycling events (he was an avid long-distance bicyclist). But although he *looked* fit and trim, he actually was exhausted. His life had become a series of endless chores, which he dutifully performed, but his joy was gone.

His regular doctor had told him, "There's nothing wrong." In fact, he had complimented Thomas on his low cholesterol and trim physique. In short, Thomas' concerns had been dismissed.

Now, as he told me the details of his past and present daily life, I listened carefully. Fatigue had crept up gradually, almost without his noticing. "I've tried to keep up my bicycling," he reported, "but I've had to cut back." It was taking longer and longer to recover the energy that he expended to keep up his pace.

Considering that his work shift varied from day to day (and even from night to night), is it any wonder that he was tired? His body could never settle into a steady rhythm. "Let's see if we can stabilize your body, to start with," I suggested. "We'll look into sleep aids so you can sleep through… whenever your sleep-time is. Also, we'll look into Vitamin B12 and support for your adrenals." (You will find more on these and other such tools a bit later in this chapter.)

"We can also work with your digestion," I went on, "including adding more good fats to your diet." (For details, see Chapter Two: "The Golden

Key—Engaging the Rhythm of Good Digestion," and Chapter Three: "Nutrition: Finding Your *Nourishing* Rhythm.")

Thomas was more than happy to collaborate with my suggestions, and as he put them into practice they helped him significantly. What's more, he changed his work schedule to a day shift, which meant waking at 4:30 a.m. in order to be at work from 7:00 a.m. to 3:30 p.m. Having a steady schedule put him on a more even keel, and he started sleeping better. However, after working together with me for six months, his fatigue was still so great that he could only tolerate about two hours of physical activity before he became exhausted.

One day, he came into my office with a resolute look in his eyes. "I'm sick and tired of being tired," he declared. "And if I have to retire early to get well, then I'll do it." This was a big decision for him. Retiring early meant less pay than if he waited another three years.

He brought his wife with him to several subsequent appointments with me, and the three of us had many conversations over the months. He came to understand that he had much more to lose than money if he stayed with his job. In my role as his doctor and advisor, I continued to support his journey and trust his own knowing of what was best for him.

> *"I'm sick and tired of being tired," he declared.*
> *"And if I have to retire early to get well, then I'll*
> *do it."*

Thomas' decision proved to be a good one. It wasn't until he decided to retire that his energy started to *fully* recover. He was able to live his life according to the Rhythms his body wanted and needed. Without the stresses and imbalances of his job, he was able to adjust his stress level to a more livable one, and returning to a regular Rhythm of sleep and awake-time made a big difference. But even with that, it took him over a year to feel like he had his old "get up and go" again.

Fourteen months after retiring, Thomas was able to return to his bicycling activities. But a month later, he reported that participating in a strenuous biking event had left him exhausted. Together, we reviewed what he was doing that wasn't working out.

"I'd been feeling so much better—what happened?" he asked. It turned out that *he had stopped taking his supplements when he began to feel good again.*

Many people make this mistake. Once the problem they originally took the supplements or medicine for has resolved, they decide that they are "cured." However, many times their body actually still needs the additional support—sometimes for years, or even a lifetime. We tend to view taking supplements and the lifestyle changes we make to improve our health like fixing a flat tire, rather than like keeping the oil level adequate in the car for the engine to run smoothly. This is not surprising in a culture that seeks quick fixes and simplistic solutions for problems that are complex and multidimensional.

Two-and-a half years after we started working on his health journey, I saw Thomas again when he accompanied his wife to *her* appointment with me. I greeted him warmly, delighted to see how good and happy he was looking. He was relaxed, and seemed actually joyful.

"You know," I confided, "I'm writing a book containing a chapter about chronic fatigue and how important it is to have a lifestyle that synchronizes with nature's diurnal Rhythm. Would you give me permission to share a bit of your experience of what it was like for you to work a schedule so out of sync with nature's Rhythms?"

He got very excited at the idea that his story might be used as an illustration, and quickly wrote down what his exact work schedule had been. "I hope this will help other air-traffic controllers," he said as he left with a big smile on his face.

For over twenty years, this was his work schedule:

- Day 1 – 4 a.m. to 12 p.m.
- Day 2 – 1 p.m. to 9 p.m.
- Day 3 – 7 a.m. to 3 p.m.
- Day 4 – 7 a.m. to 3 p.m.
- Day 5 – 11 p.m. to 7 a.m. (starting 9 hours after his previous shift)
- Days 6 and 7 – off

Can you imagine? Who would *not* be affected by having to recalibrate and reboot over and over and over? Fortunately, he had been able to see how his work-lifestyle was sabotaging his health and to make the decision to live more naturally and fully.

The old adage "early to bed, early to rise…" has a grain of wisdom in it, honoring the importance of synchronizing with nature's rhythm of day and night, activity and rest. When our own rhythms harmonize with nature's, we are supported. We're not fighting the tides—we can flow *with* them, and life becomes easeful, savored, and joyful.

Although this was not remotely Thomas's situation for all the years he worked such erratic hours, it *became* his situation once he retired and started living in harmony with his natural Rhythms.

EACH PERSON'S FATIGUE IS A UNIQUE STORY

For me as a health professional, it takes time—often, several hours—to hear a patient's entire story. Only then can I begin to put the pieces together and get a clearer understanding of the natural history of each person's fatigue.

Some people can remember exactly when it started—perhaps after a specific illness, or childbirth, or the death of a loved one. Others remember that even as a child, they were less active and more easily tired than other children, and needed more sleep. Some people are not sure when it started. It seemed to creep up on them imperceptibly. And still others have been maintaining a lifestyle that would burn out Wonder Woman or Superman.

The CDC (Centers for Disease Control and Prevention) has defined Chronic Fatigue Syndrome as having these symptoms:

All of the following:

- Severe chronic fatigue for over six consecutive months that is not due to ongoing exertion or other medical conditions associated with fatigue.

- The fatigue significantly interferes with daily activities and/or work.

Four or more of the following eight symptoms *concurrently*:

- Unrefreshing sleep.

- Post-exertion malaise lasting more than 24 hours.

- Muscle pain.

▪ Multi-joint pain without swelling or redness.

▪ Headaches of a new type, pattern, or severity.

▪ Tender cervical or axillary lymph nodes.

▪ Sore throat that is frequent or recurring.

The term "Chronic Fatigue Syndrome" (CFS) is, as I said at the start of this chapter, basically a waste-basket term. It is used by doctors to mean, "We believe you are really tired, and we don't know the reason why." Being given the diagnosis of CFS in itself does not help you to figure out what is the *cause* of the fatigue, nor help you determine how to best *resolve* it.

There *are* lab tests that can help to identify possible contributors to chronic fatigue. Standard blood tests, such as a CBC (see the Glossary for an explanation) can help rule out anemia from iron, folate, or B12-deficiency, or the very rare possibility of leukemia. But by the time I see a patient, these tests most often have already been done and those illnesses have been ruled out. The usual blood tests that most doctors order do not fully evaluate some of the *other* common sources of chronic fatigue, such as thyroid and adrenal dysfunction.

THYROID PROBLEMS

Thyroid problems affect women four times as frequently as men. Typically, the first sign that a woman notices is a change in her energy level.

Remember my patient Soraya (described in Chapter Three: "Nutrition—Finding Your *Nourishing* Rhythm"), who complained of low energy? She returned to see me after a month on a low-carbohydrate, high-fat meal plan.

"I've lost some weight and I am definitely feeling better," she reported. "But I still don't have the energy I used to have. I've done some reading, and I think my problem is my thyroid."

"When did you first notice feeling tired or low-energy?" I inquired. Getting the full history about her fatigue would be key to figuring out the root cause.

"It seems like it started after my second baby was born. I just never bounced back. And that's also when the weight started to pile on," Soraya reflected. "I thought it might be my thyroid."

Thyroid problems affect women four times as frequently as men. They often begin when there is a big shift in estrogen hormone levels. Estrogen levels make dramatic shifts in women at puberty, pregnancy, post-partum, and menopause. Like Soraya, many women can track when they first noted a major change in their energy to one of these times. Typically, the first sign that a woman notices is a change in her energy level. She is much more tired. She may also notice that she sleeps more, feels cold, is constipated, may feel puffy, gains weight, her hair may thin and her nails are weak—and overall, she just doesn't feel like her previous self.

"I've had my thyroid checked several times," Soraya continued, "and the doctors always said it was fine."

I could hear frustration in her voice. She had probably been telling her doctors that she was tired for years.

"Do you have a copy of any recent thyroid tests that I could see?" I asked her.

She shook her head. "No, sorry," she answered. "And I can't remember what was checked out."

*"I've had my thyroid checked several times,"
Soraya said, "and the doctors always said it was
fine." I could hear frustration in her voice. She had
probably been telling her doctors that she was tired
for years.*

Then she added, "Did I tell you that my *mother* had a thyroid problem? I *still* think I have a thyroid problem too."

My sense was that she probably was right. *Many* patients with fatigue have an undiagnosed thyroid problem. Often, they've had their thyroid "checked" and been told, "There's nothing wrong." And, like Soraya, they often have a history of others in their family having thyroid issues, such as Hashimoto's hypothyroid or hyperthyroid, or Graves Disease, or goiters.

What Is the Thyroid?

To understand the physiology of what happens when there is a thyroid problem, let's look at the thyroid gland itself.

The thyroid is an endocrine gland located in the neck. It is one of the glands responsible for setting our metabolic rate—our energy level. An under-functioning thyroid (*hypo*thyroidism) can certainly be a cause of chronic fatigue. Untreated hypothyroidism can contribute to hypertension, elevated cholesterol, infertility, cognitive impairment, neuromuscular dysfunction, and a host of other symptoms.

The thyroid gland produces a thyroid hormone called T4, which stimulates metabolism. T4 is converted to T3 in the body. T3 is about four times stronger than T4. The hypothalamus is the part of the brain that governs the level of TSH, or Thyroid Stimulating Hormone. When it perceives the levels of T4 and T3 in the blood, it signals the pituitary gland to make TSH. The level of TSH controls the production of thyroid hormone. A high TSH stimulates the thyroid gland to make *more* T4. If there is very little TSH, the thyroid gland will make *less* T4.

Why Do So Many Doctors Fail to Diagnose Thyroid Problems?

When doctors order lab tests to check a patient's thyroid, the standard blood test that most of them use is the TSH. If the test results show that the patient's TSH level is in the laboratory range for "normal," most doctors will tell the patient, "There is no problem with your thyroid"—even if it is barely in the normal range and the patient has many hypothyroid symptoms. A number of patients have told me of having experiences like this. No wonder they are frustrated!

> *If the test results show that the patient's TSH level is in the laboratory range for "normal," most doctors will tell the patient, "There is no problem with your thyroid"—even if it is barely in the normal range and the patient has many hypothyroid symptoms.*

Here's the difficulty, as I see it: when the test for TSH was originally developed, doctors then needed to establish the range of normal values for TSH. So they chose a hundred people whom they deemed to be normal, and obtained *their* TSH levels. The TSH range of "normal" was created from those values, and this is the criterion that's still used today. When your TSH is checked, the laboratory reports the number for your TSH level, and gives the range of normal as being 0.0450 - 4.500 mIU/L (with slight variation, depending on the lab).

There have been recommendations to revise this criterion of "normal." For instance, in 2003, the American Association of Clinical Endocrinologists recommended that the TSH range of normal be lowered to .3 - 3.0 mIU/L. If the labs used this range of normal, many more hypothyroid conditions would be diagnosed. Unfortunately, however, many doctors (including some endocrinologists) are not acting on this recommendation. Then in 2012, the Clinical Practice Guidelines for Hypothyroidism in Adults (cosponsored by the American Association of Clinical Endocrinologists and the American Thyroid Association) recommended that 4.12 mIU/L be viewed as the upper limit of "normal" for TSH. Even so, most laboratories still use the old TSH normal range of 0.4 - 4.4 mIU/L.

Confused? It is *very* confusing. No wonder so many people with hypothyroidism go undiagnosed!

And so, to address Soraya's concerns, I told her, "I suggest that we do a full work-up of your thyroid function. A 'full work-up' includes checking levels of TSH, free T4, free T3, reverse T3, thyroid peroxidase antibody (TPO), and antithyroglobulin antibody. We should also check your iodine levels," I added, "because iodine is needed to convert T4 to T3."

"Finally!" Soraya exclaimed. "Someone in the medical profession who *listens* to me! I've been asking doctors to do some of these tests for years, but they refuse to do anything different."

> *"Finally! Someone in the medical profession who listens to me!"*

Moments like this make my heart sing. Here was someone who finally felt heard and validated for her self-awareness and skillful reasoning. It makes me sad to hear so many stories of patients who are told that they don't have a problem, that nothing is wrong, or even that perhaps they are fatuously wasting their doctor's time.

I have seen a number of patients who began doing their own research to get some answers. They read books such as *Overcoming Thyroid Disorders*,

Stop the Thyroid Madness, and *Why Am I So Tired?* as well as searching the Internet. Although they are quite certain that their fatigue is thyroid-related, they cannot find a doctor who is willing to treat them—all because their TSH is within the normal range. These people have many of the symptoms of an under-functioning thyroid, such as hair loss, thin skin, constipation, being frequently sick and slow to recover, low blood pressure, low body temperature, a history of miscarriages, feeling cold, and many more.

"I have had my T4 levels checked and been told it was normal!" Soraya sounded very frustrated. "How can it be normal when I feel so bad?"

"The thyroid gland makes a hormone called T4," I explained, "which the body converts into a hormone called T3. T3 is four times as powerful as T4. Some doctors do check the levels of T4, but not T3. They aren't checking to see if the body is able to *convert* T4 to T3. Remember, T3 is four times more potent than T4."

If a person is already taking thyroid medication such as Synthroid or a generic of it, such as levoxyl or levothyroxine, they are taking synthetic T4. Checking for the hormone levels of T4 in blood tests only checks for the hormone that they are supplementing with medication.

Even doctors who check the levels of b*oth* T3 and T4 often miss the boat, because they are checking the *total* hormone levels, not the *levels of free hormone*. That is, they fail to check the levels of the *free T3* and *free T4*. The free hormone is the part that is *available* to bind to the thyroid hormone receptor sites. It is also important to check *Reverse T3*, an inactive form of T3. Sometimes the body shunts T4 into Reverse T3 instead of into the active form of T3. (It may do this for various reasons, including to keep metabolism low as a protective measure.)

The typical thyroid testing that most doctors undertake is another example of looking for the lost keys under the street light rather than searching the dark part of the street where they actually were lost. And the standard Thyroid Function Panel that the major laboratories offer does not check the *free* levels of hormones T4 and T3, nor Reverse T3, nor the thyroid antibodies.

"Let's do a thorough test of your thyroid function," I suggested to Soraya. "We'll check the TSH, free T4 and free T3, reverse T3, and also levels of the thyroid antibodies and iodine. That should give us a good picture of what is going on." She agreed, and left her appointment very excited.

When the blood-test results came back, Soraya returned, and we reviewed her blood work together. It turned out that her T4 levels were in the normal range, but her T3 was quite low. "You make plenty of T4, but it is not being converted into sufficient quantities of T3," I explained as we jointly looked at the results. "That indicates a T4-to-T3 conversion dysfunction, so giving you more T4 won't solve the problem." This explains why taking additional synthetic T4, whether Synthroid or generic, doesn't help some people feel better.

"Your iodine levels are good," I told her, "but the body also needs *selenium*, and the amino acid *tyrosine* to convert T4 to T3." I could see that Soraya was following me closely as she looked at the numbers and the simple pictures I drew to explain the process.

In general, with those patients for whom T4-to-T3-conversion is a problem, there are a number of ways that I have found helpful to improve the process.

- If *iodine* is low, supplemental iodine, or adding seaweed such as dulse or kelp to your diet, can be helpful.

- Low *tyrosine* may be from a low-protein diet or a lack of sufficient digestive enzymes to break down and absorb proteins.

- There are also supplements available that contain all three: iodine, selenium, and tyrosine.

"Let's look at your options," I continued. "We could try a supplement that contains tyrosine, iodine, and selenium. Another option is to add actual T3. A third option is to add both the thyroid hormones T4 and T3. Both T3 and the combination T3-and-T4 are prescription medications, although some thyroid glandulars are available over the counter."

I trust that the best solution is the one that my patient will choose, guided by my information and support. Improving thyroid function is often a matter of trying different solutions until the one that works best can be found. I tend to follow my patients' intuition or "gut feeling" about which approach to try first. I want to build their confidence that they can correctly assess the benefit for themselves, as well as grow their trust in me as a supportive member of their team.

"I think I would like to try the supplement that boosts T4-to-T3 conversion first," Soraya declared. "I would rather not start with taking extra thyroid hormone." And so we agreed to a two-month trial period. At that point, she would get her blood retested, then return for an appointment with me to report on how she was doing.

After two months, Soraya returned to see me. "My energy is somewhat better, but still not where I would like it to be," she reported.

We looked at her most recent blood tests together. "Your new lab test results show that levels of free T3 and free T4 are both in the bottom third of the normal range," I told her. "I think taking additional thyroid hormone may be helpful. Why don't we do a trial for two or three months and see how you feel?"

But at this, Soraya looked troubled. "I'm afraid that if I start taking thyroid hormone now, I'll have to take it for the rest of my life!"

"Some patients have that worry because this is what they have been told," I reassured her. "However, I have seen some patients who took thyroid hormone for a period of months or even years, and then no longer needed to take it."

"Perhaps, after some time, their own thyroid gland recovered and was able to function better?" Soraya was puzzled.

I nodded. "And some patients seem to need more thyroid hormone in the winter and less during the summer. Some people experience an improvement in energy using homeopathic thyroid products, alone. And there are some who need less or no hormone, once the thyroid antibodies disappear. "

Telling Soraya this seemed to calm her anxiety. But she also had strong feelings about what she did *not* want to take. "I don't want to take Synthroid or the generic levothyroxine. My mom has taken it for years, and she says she doesn't feel any better." Soraya clearly had already done some investigating.

The thyroid medications that she mentioned—*Synthroid,* or its generic, *levothyroxine* or *levoxyl*—have been taken for years by a number of patients diagnosed as "hypothyroid" who later came to see me. These patients hadn't felt any better, or at best were only slightly improved. Many times, they had returned to their doctor and complained, but their doctors told them that their levels were normal and refused to change the medication. And their hypothyroid symptoms persisted.

"I can understand why you don't want to take Synthroid," I responded. "When patients taking it come to me because they still don't feel right, we try the *porcine thyroid* prescription. Most of the patients who took this feel significantly better on it. Many began to feel for the first time after many years—like their old selves."

There *are* alternatives to Synthroid and levothyroxine or levoxyl. Most people suffering from hypothyroidism usually notice a significant improvement when they switch to a thyroid hormone product made from porcine (pig) thyroid. *Armour Thyroid*, *Nature-Thyroid*, and *Westhroid* are all prescription thyroid-hormone compounds made from USP desiccated porcine thyroid ("USP" is a standardized prescription dose monitored by the FDA). They contain a combination of T4 *and* T3, as well as other elements found in the pig's thyroid gland. These prescription medications are available in any pharmacy. In my experience, about 70 percent of the people with an under-functioning thyroid find that the porcine thyroid products are much more effective than Synthroid or other synthetic T4 products.

"What if I just took some additional T3?" Soraya asked curiously.

"Some people have been given additional prescription T3 by their doctor," I confirmed. "This is a synthetic product and has about a four-hour half-life. This means that it needs to be taken several times a day to maintain an adequate level of T3." I added, "I have found the porcine thyroid products to be as effective, in most cases. And you don't need to take it as often."

"Well, that makes sense to me. But when I asked the doctor to pre-scribe Armour thyroid for my mother," Soraya reported, "I was told that it was unreliable and not safe, and should never be used."

"Yes, I know." I found myself nodding sympathetically. "Back when I was in medical school, we were taught that we should only prescribe the synthetic T4 product Synthroid. We were told that the amount of thyroid hormone in the porcine product could vary widely and be dangerous."

Soraya's eyebrows rose slightly.

I reassured her, "That may have been true at one time many years ago, but not today. Over the years, I have followed hundreds of people who switched to Armour thyroid or one of the other prescription porcine-thyroid products, and none of them has ever had a problem with experiencing adverse effects from uneven dosage."

After discussing her options together, Soraya and I decided to start a trial of porcine thyroid. "We will start with the smallest amount and gradually increase it each month," I advised.

"How will I know if it's too much?"

"It is fairly easy to tell if you are taking too high a dose," I told her. "Too much thyroid hormone feels a lot like too much caffeine. You may experience palpitations, or heart thumps or pounding, or chest tightness; or there may be tremors, irritability, or difficulty sleeping. If any of these symptoms occur, just stop taking the thyroid hormone until the symptoms subside, and then go back to your previous lower dose."

Hashimoto's Thyroiditis

Then Soraya surprised me by asking, "Do I have Hashimoto's hypothyroid? I've been reading about it." She certainly was engaged in her own healing process.

Hashimoto's Thyroiditis is a hypothyroid condition in which the body makes antibodies to thyroid tissue. If someone has high levels of thyroid antibodies, it means that these are interfering with thyroid function. Therefore, it is important to bring those levels down. The presence of antibodies also indicates that there is some inflammation in the thyroid.

"When we tested you for thyroid antibodies such as thyroid peroxidase antibody and anti-thyroglobulin antibody," I told her, "we found that your levels were high. So, yes, you do have Hashimoto's thyroiditis." To put her more at ease, I added, "It's very common."

Soraya looked worried. "Is there anything I can do about it?"

"Yes, actually, there is," I replied.

I could see her face relax.

"Often," I explained, "people with high levels of thyroid antibodies have a lot of inflammation in other areas of their bodies, as well. One of the most helpful ways to significantly reduce inflammation is to remove gluten from your diet."

"Gluten?" she repeated.

"Going gluten-free can help reduce the amount of thyroid antibodies. Gluten-rich grains increase inflammation and need to be avoided. These grains include wheat, rye, barley, oats, triticale, spelt, and kamut." I gave her a handout listing the high-gluten grains and the low-gluten grains.

(For more details on the effect of gluten, see Chapter Two: The Golden Key—Engaging the Rhythms of Good Digestion," and Chapter Three: "Nutrition—Finding Your *Nourishing* Rhythm.")

"Anything else?" she asked me.

"Removing sugar is also helpful."

At this, Soraya laughed. "I've already started doing that with my low-carbohydrate diet. But why does it matter for the thyroid?"

I decided that more explanation was needed. "Sugar is a very inflammatory food. By 'sugar,' I don't mean the sugar that naturally occurs in foods, like lactose sugar in milk. I mean *added sugar*, such as sucrose, fructose, glucose, and others listed as 'ingredients' on product labels. If we want to reduce thyroid antibody levels, it's important to reduce inflammatory foods as much as possible." I repeated the reasoning, hoping Soraya could see the importance.

"OK," she sighed. "I've probably had enough cookies and donuts to last me the rest of my life. I'm willing to make those changes if it will make me feel better."

For some people, removing other foods that they are reactive to can help reduce overall inflammation. Food sensitivities and allergies cause a lot of inflammation in the body. (See Chapter Three: "Nutrition—Finding Your *Nourishing* Rhythm" for further details.)

"Another way to reduce thyroid antibody levels is to *alkalinize* the body," I explained, "Most people have a body pH of around 5.0, which is quite acid. In order to alkalinize, they need to choose more of the foods that are alkaline, and fewer of the acid-forming foods."

"How do I tell if a food is alkaline or acid?" Soraya wanted to know.

"In general, processed foods are much more acidic, and most vegetables are more alkaline. A simple way is to eat lots more vegetables and cut out processed foods."

"How will I know if it's working?"

"You can use pH strips or tape and test the alkalinity of your first morning's urine," I told her. "Your goal is a pH between 6.4 and 7.6. I have seen people reduce their thyroid antibody count by increasing the amounts of leafy vegetables and other alkaline foods in their diet, and reducing the amount of highly acidic foods, such as sugar and white flour."

I gave her a chart that listed foods in categories from "Most Alkaline" to "Most Acid." (See the Appendix, Chapter Nine, for a copy of this chart.)

Soraya looked a bit overwhelmed, which was understandable. I had given her a lot of new information, and was suggesting that she make some fundamental dietary changes. To encourage her, I reminded her, "You'll be able to do it! You have already eliminated a lot of inflammatory foods by changing your diet and eating low-carbohydrate organic foods." I felt like her midwife, encouraging her in her labor as she hit a difficult moment.

I added, "Another approach is to take buffered Vitamin C to alkalinize the body. This method was developed by Dr. Russell Jaffee, an immunologist. It usually takes at least six months of being off gluten and keeping an alkaline pH to see a significant decrease in the thyroid antibodies. However, it can be worth it. I have seen some people reduce their thyroid antibodies to zero." (The Ascorbate Flush and protocol developed by Dr. Jaffee are in the Appendix, Chapter Nine.)

Soraya didn't seem interested in taking on the alkaline protocol at this time. "I've decided to try the porcine thyroid!" she smiled. "I can't wait to feel better. And I'm willing to avoid gluten and sugar."

But I felt obliged to break into her enthusiasm by cautioning her, "Before we start you on any thyroid hormone, we need to check your adrenal function."

"Why is that?" She looked quizzical.

"When I first started using the porcine thyroid with hypothyroid patients who experienced fatigue," I explained, "I noticed that sometimes these patients felt remarkably better—at first. But then, about three to six months later, they crashed and were back experiencing their old fatigue again. That was before I learned that energy and metabolism are the responsibility of *two* glands: the thyroid…"

Soraya nodded.

"… and two tiny glands situated on the kidneys called the *adrenal glands*."

THE ADRENAL GLANDS

I like to think of the thyroid and the adrenals as two big Clydesdale horses hitched to our Energy Wagon. If the thyroid horse has not been pulling its weight, the adrenal horse has had to pick up the extra load in order to keep up the pace. Over time, the overworked adrenal horse may also become fatigued and unable to maintain the pace. At this point, we experience fatigue because neither the thyroid *nor* the adrenals are able to keep up with the demand for energy.

When we add extra thyroid hormone, we are whipping up the thyroid horse. However, if the adrenal horse also has become weak, now the *thyroid* must pull the extra load. It can do this for a while, but eventually the additional burden will overwhelm it and it will no longer be able to keep up the pace. This is what happened when my patients' fatigue recurred after starting porcine thyroid. The fatigue results because both the adrenal *and* the thyroid glands are unable to maintain a good output of hormone. They both are functioning sub-optimally, if at all.

So from experience, I have learned that if fatigue is an issue, the health of the adrenal glands *as well as* the thyroid must be checked. And if they both are not functioning optimally, it is vital that both be supported to avoid subsequent crashes in energy.

> *If fatigue is an issue, the health of the adrenal glands as well as the thyroid must be checked, and—if not functionally optimally—be supported.*

What Is Adrenal Fatigue?

In medical school, I was taught about a condition called Addison's Disease. Since then, I have learned that Addison's Disease really is just the end stage of adrenal fatigue—when the adrenals have completely stopped functioning. At that point, they are no longer making any adrenal hormones, which include *cortisol, DHEA,* and *aldosterone.*

But just as we can observe that a horse is getting tired well before it drops dead of exhaustion, we can also detect adrenal fatigue well before it fails completely—*if* we know what to look for. What I wasn't taught in medical school was that there are *degrees* of adrenal exhaustion, and how to detect, evaluate, and treat them before the adrenals completely stop working.

"How would I know if my adrenals aren't working well?" Soraya was curious.

"Adrenal fatigue can have some of the same symptoms as hypothyroidism," I explained to her, "including fatigue, feeling cold, being frequently sick and slow to recover—but it also has unique symptoms that are different from hypothyroidism. These symptoms include fatigue that becomes worse after exercise or strenuous activity; a decreased libido; needing to wear sunglasses a lot because bright light bothers the eyes; brain fog or mental confusion when very tired; anxiety; disturbed sleep; and depression."

Tapping the knees with a reflex hammer can tell a lot. A person with *simple hypothyroidism* will have rather sluggish reflexes, especially the Achilles-tendon reflex. A person with pur*e adrenal fatigue* will have hyper-responsive knee reflexes. (If a person has both adrenal and thyroid dysfunction, then the reflex response can be mixed and harder to interpret.)

"Do you usually wear sunglasses?" I asked Soraya.

"I wear them pretty much all the time when I'm outside, even in the winter. Why did you ask?"

"It can be another sign that your adrenals are fatigued," I explained. "The pupils of the eye are supposed to constrict in bright light. This reflex is controlled by the adrenal hormone, cortisol. If the adrenals are unable to mount an adequate cortisol response, the pupils can't stay constricted and so bright light is uncomfortable."

A good test of pupillary response is to shine a bright light into the eyes of a person. (This test works best in a darkened room.) If the adrenals are weak, the pupils will attempt to constrict in response to the light but will be unable to hold the constriction. You will see the pupil growing larger and smaller, larger and smaller over and over, because the lack of cortisol production makes the pupils unable to hold the constriction. Sometimes the pupils will constrict for less than a second and then remain large.

One of my most severely adrenally depleted patients, Connie, recently told me that she thought she already had adrenal problems as a child. She remembered lying in her bed, looking at headlights of cars passing outside in the streets and enjoying how the headlights rhythmically grew bigger and smaller, bigger and smaller as she looked. It was a source of entertainment for her at that time. Little did she know that it also was a clue to her weakened adrenal state.

Another sign of adrenal fatigue is when the pads of the fingertips develop vertical lines, something like the "prune fingers" that develop after staying in water too long. Loss of hair, both scalp and pubic, and sallow complexion can also be signs of adrenal fatigue.

"How do we test my adrenals?" Soraya was eager to learn.

I pulled out a piece of paper and sketched a simple graph with a line that started high on the left and drifted to its lowest point on the far right. "We test for the adrenal hormones cortisol and DHEA. Cortisol production has a diurnal cycle. When the adrenals are functioning well, the highest level of cortisol is produced in the morning, and the amount slowly decreases over the day, with the lowest levels occurring at night. Our bodies are meant to be in harmony with nature, waking us up with the morning sun with 'get-up-and-go!' energy from a high cortisol level, and allowing us restful sleep at night when cortisol is at its lowest level.

"The best way to test both the amount and timing of cortisol output during the 24-hour-cycle," I explained to her, "is to collect multiple saliva samples throughout the day. Cortisol can be tested in the saliva, so you don't need a blood test. I usually check cortisol levels at four specific times: early morning, noon, late afternoon, and late at night. I use saliva samples because they are easy for the patient to collect."

I brought out a saliva test kit and explained to Soraya how to collect her saliva to be tested for cortisol. "Be sure you don't use any caffeine or stimulants on the day you collect the saliva. After you collect each sample, label it with the time you collected it and put it in the fridge." Depending on which lab we chose, she would drop it in the mail or deliver it to the lab the next day.

"After we see what your pattern and quantity of cortisol output is, we can tell if your problem is a rhythm problem, a total output problem, or some combination of both," I concluded.

Adrenal problems having to do with cortisol can be a rhythm problem, a total output problem, or a combination of both.

If Soraya's cortisol was lowest in the morning and highest at night, that would be a *rhythm* problem. It would indicate that the adrenals can produce enough cortisol, but the output is not synchronized with the day/night cycle. If her levels of cortisol were low at all the collection times, then she would have an *output* problem: the adrenals simply cannot make enough cortisol. As you can see, the information obtained from collecting at four different times during the 24-hour cycle is much more helpful than just a random or morning blood-cortisol level.

DHEA is another hormone that's produced by the adrenals. It is concerned with repair and restorative function. One can test for DHEA with saliva or with a blood test for DHEA-sulfate (DHEA-S), a breakdown product of DHEA. If either DHEA or DHEA-sulfate is low, this can indicate a lack of adrenal reserves. Some labs can also test the level of precursor molecules such as pregnenolone and 17-hydroxyprogesterone. If these precursors are depleted, then that may help explain why cortisol or DHEA levels are low.

When Soraya returned a week later to review the results of her cortisol test, we looked at the graph. All the values, even the early-morning levels, were low. As I explained the graph and numbers to Soraya, she began to look alarmed.

"So if my adrenals are weak, what does that mean? Is there anything we can do to improve them?"

"It means," I explained, "that we need to support the *adrenals* as well as the thyroid in order for your energy to return to your normal feel-good levels. Remember my comparison of the thyroid and adrenals as two big plow horses pulling your energy wagon?"

Soraya nodded vigorously, still looking worried.

"Your thyroid probably has been under-functioning since you had your second baby. The adrenals have had to pull more than their share of the load for quite a while. At some point, they reached their limit and became weak. If we just whip the thyroid horse with hormones, it will have to pull more than its share because the adrenals are now weak. So it is only a matter of time before they cannot continue—and you will know it, because your energy will become low again. That's why we have to support them *both* in order for you to fully recover."

"I think I understand what you're saying. So it's good we tested the adrenals before I started taking thyroid hormone?"

"Yes. Before I understood about the adrenals, I used to start people on thyroid hormone and they felt great for a while. Then, after around three to six months, their energy would tank again. I couldn't understand why, then; but now I do, so I check both thyroid and adrenals and get much better results."

I went on to explain to Soraya that there are many ways to boost overall adrenal function.

Herbs

Herbs are very effective in supporting and rebuilding the adrenals. Every culture or healing tradition has its favorite restorative herb, such as the Ayurvedic herb Ashwagandha (*Withania somnifera*), the Western herbal medicine Eleutherococcus senticosus, and Chinese medicine's Panax ginseng, among others. In addition, there are many other herbs that have proven very helpful for the adrenals, such as licorice and rhodiola.

BOOST ADRENAL FUNCTION BY:

- **Using restorative herbs**
  Ashwagandha
  Eleutherococcus senticosus
  Panax ginseng
  Licorice
  Rhodiola

- **A good (alkalinizing) diet**
  Fruits
  Veggies
  Saturated fats
  Less sugar, simple carbs
  B vitamins
  Minerals
  Sea salt

Diet

A good diet is very important—one with plenty of fruits and vegetables to alkalinize the body, adequate amounts of saturated fats (at least 30 percent of one's daily calories), and reduced intake of sugar and simple carbohydrates. Large amounts of B vitamins, adequate mineral support, and liberal use of sea salt helps, as well.

Sleep

Getting refreshing sleep in adequate amounts is vital for recovery. The average adult really does need eight hours of sleep. Six hours a night is just not enough for most people. In the winter months, with the longer nights and shorter days, we often need even more sleep.

Cultivating natural sleep-rhythms: What we observe in nature is that living creatures have shorter periods of activity in the wintertime. Some completely hibernate, and some go dormant. Unfortunately, in our culture, the lifestyle of the natural world is mostly unnoticed or seen as irrelevant. Few of us spend enough time in nature to observe the seasonal changes closely. Thanks to electric lights, we can ignore the reduced daylight of a winter day. School schedules and most people's work schedules do not make seasonal adjustments.

Where I live, many people spend winter months getting up in the dark and coming home in the dark. No wonder so many people are sick in January! They spent December ignoring the growing darkness and attending parties and events late into the night. Maybe we could learn to party the Scandinavian way. Friends have told me of New Year's Eve parties there that went on for three days, partying by day and sleeping through the long nights. Sounds like fun without the drain.

It has been said that sleep during the hours before midnight is *golden*. If at all possible, try to get at least two hours of sleep in before midnight. Some people with adrenal fatigue find an *afternoon nap* of about 30 to 90 minutes to be very helpful, as long as it doesn't detract from their ability to sleep at night. This nap should be taken between 2 and 4 p.m.

Good sleep hygiene: Most people are familiar by now with what has been termed *good sleep hygiene*. These are factors known to be helpful for inducing restful sleep. They include:

- Keep the bedroom as dark as possible.

- Eliminate TV, radio, nightlights, streetlights, clock dials and other electronic devices from the bedroom. Many electronic devices—such as computer screens, Kindles, and cell phones—emit light in the blue wave-frequency. The blue frequency is stimulating to the brain.

- Avoid using any electronics after 9 p.m. or an hour before you plan to go to bed.

- Read in bed using a *real* book or magazine.

Insomnia: *Insomnia* is a broad term and doesn't really clarify what the specific type of sleep problem is. Some people have difficulty falling asleep. Others fall asleep easily but cannot *stay* asleep, and wake up hour after hour. Still others awaken only in the wee hours of the morning and can't get back to sleep until after dawn. Each of these sleep problems has different causes and different solutions.

Some people aren't sleeping because their cortisol is highest at night, when it should be lowest. Taking 500mg or more of the amino acid phosphatidylserine at bedtime or an hour before can be helpful. It lowers cortisol levels by increasing the liver's ability to break it down and remove it from circulation.

If elevated cortisol at night is not the reason for sleep difficulties, there are other approaches worth trying.

- There are herbs that help one *relax*, like Hops and Valerian, and there are others that soothe and rebuild the nerves, like Passionflower and Milky Oat Seed.

- The homeopathic remedy *Coffea cruda* helps if you can't fall asleep because your mind just keeps on racing (as if you had drunk too much coffee), even though your body feels tired.

> **INCUBATING GOOD SLEEP:**
>
> Get to sleep before midnight (by 10 p.m., preferably)
>
> ✦
>
> Consider napping (between 2-4 p.m. is ideal)
>
> ✦
>
> Keep your bedroom dark
>
> ✦
>
> Eliminate all electronic devices from the bedroom
>
> ✦
>
> Don't use any electronics after 9 p.m. or an hour before bed
>
> ✦
>
> If you like to read in bed, make it a (physical) book or magazine

- Melatonin taken at bedtime is helpful to reset the sleep-wake cycle. The pineal gland normally secretes melatonin at night. Some people with adrenal fatigue have problems with their hypothalamic-pituitary axis and melatonin production. Start with a very low dose of melatonin, such as 1mg, and add more if that is not enough.

- CBD, a component of cannabis, can be taken just before bedtime

- Sometimes a prescription sleeping medication is necessary to help reinstate a sleep-wake cycle that is coordinated with the day-night cycle.

People who work night-shift jobs can find it difficult to keep adjusting their body Rhythms from sleeping *days* when they work, to sleeping *nights* on their days off. Most difficult of all are jobs that continually rotate shifts, like air-traffic control (remember Thomas?). These people might work two weeks on the morning shift, then two weeks on swing shift, and then two weeks on night shift, and repeat. Many nurses, police, and fire-department employees work shift jobs. Their bodies never have a chance to settle into a long period of unchanging diurnal cycle, and it can have a significant effect on their long-term health.

Supplements, Prescriptions, and Other Therapeutic Modalities

In addition to lifestyle and dietary interventions, there are supplements that can help support rebuilding the adrenals. Taking an adrenal glandular containing

To Help with Insomnia and Adrenal Fatigue:

If your cortisol is high at night, take 500+ mg of phosphatidylserine.

Take **Melatonin** (start with a low dose, increase if needed).

Herbs can help. Consider:
Hops
Valerian
Passionflower
Milky Oat Seed
CBD

Homeopathic remedies—*Coffea cruda*

Supplements—consider:
Adrenal-glandulars (e.g., from Standard Process, American Biologics, Biotics, Thorne)

Prescriptions—Cortef

Other therapeutic modalities to consider:
Acupuncture
Polarity therapy
Reflexology
Cranio-sacral therapy

adrenal-gland material from animals is often helpful. This can provide the additional energy needed while the adrenals are healing. There are many different companies making these. I recommend reputable sources such as Standard Process, American Biologics, Biotics, or Thorne.

Adding a prescription hydrocortisone—a synthetic cortisol called Cortef—can be another source of energy. Do not confuse Cortef with prednisone. Cortef is much weaker than prednisone and is used in adrenal fatigue to bring cortisol levels up to a normal physiologic range. It is important not to increase cortisol levels *beyond* the normal range. Super-physiologic levels can be harmful and counterproductive for weak adrenals. Prednisone is typically used at supra-physiological levels as a heroic measure to suppress inflammation, and should be used with great caution.

Many people use a combination of approaches, finding what works best for them. Other therapeutic modalities that I have seen help adrenal fatigue include acupuncture, polarity therapy, reflexology, and cranio-sacral therapy.

Salt Matters

"By the way," I asked Soraya, "do you salt your food?"

"I use very little salt when I cook. And I don't add any at the table. Why do you ask?"

"Because salt—by which I mean *natural sea salt*—is a key ingredient to supporting the adrenals," I told her. I could almost anticipate her next response.

"But I've always heard that salt is *bad* for you!" Soraya protested, looking even more puzzled. "Even my doctor has told me to cut back on salt. And my parents avoided salt because of my dad's blood pressure, so I'm not used to even having it around."

I answered her, "Many people have virtually eliminated salt from their diet under the misconception that salt is bad for health. But the reality is that we *need salt*. The need for salt is even supported historically: it created the earliest trade routes in human history. So the idea that salt is bad for you really is a myth."

Soraya's jaw dropped at this. "My doctor even told me to reduce my salt intake because of my blood pressure!"

"Yes, many doctors, as well as other people, still believe that myth." I shook my head. "But salt doesn't raise your blood pressure—unless you're one of the tiny minority of people who actually *swells* when they eat salt, even the small amount that's in a dill pickle. And I don't get the sense that you are."

Soraya shook her head "no."

I continued, "Many people find themselves craving salty snacks like chips and pretzels. This craving is their body telling them that they need *more* salt. I often recommend that people change from drinking plain water to water with a pinch of salt. If you are sweating a lot, you can also add a little coconut water for additional potassium, together with the salt. This is a refreshing, electrolyte-rich drink that will support your body's needs much better than plain water. If you don't have enough time to make the drink every day, at least put a pinch of salt in your drinking water."

IF YOU CRAVE SALTY SNACKS:

Add a pinch of salt to your drinking water.

(And maybe a bit of coconut water, too)

Together, Soraya and I decided on a number of interventions to improve her adrenals. I gave her a tincture of herbs that included ashwagandha, licorice, and eleutherococcus. I also gave her some phosphatidylserine to take before bed. She left my office with a written outline of her new regimen, as well as a prescription for porcine thyroid hormone.

Adrenal Healing Can Take Time

When Soraya returned a few months later, I asked her eagerly, "How is your energy, these days?"

"I'm about 60 percent better," she said. "I'm sleeping better, and I have more energy during the day. But I still tank around 3 p.m. How long will it take for my adrenals to fully recover?"

"It can take a while," I admitted, hoping that this wouldn't discourage her. "Usually, people can feel some improvement within a few weeks.

However, typically it can take six months to a year—sometimes longer—to fully recover."

Soraya's face kept its hopeful look, but her mouth turned down at the corners for just a moment.

"I know this isn't easy," I acknowledged. "And you deserve to be congratulated for coming as far as you have. You are really on a hero's journey, you know." I often feel like my patients' cheerleader, and yet I don't want to encourage false expectations. Above all, I don't want to lose their trust.

"Well, okay," Soraya rallied. "You're right. I've come this far, I can hang in until I'm fully recovered." And she left my office much more encouraged.

Remember Connie, my patient who had fun as a child watching car headlights grow larger and smaller? She had suffered from some level of adrenal fatigue since childhood. By the time she was in her forties, she was virtually unable to get off the couch. And with four kids to manage, that made life tough. But four years later, after customized treatment, she reported that she has enough energy to be active and even exercise moderately. She still needs to make sure she gets enough sleep, though—which, for her, means ten hours a night.

For many people, making the kind of *rhythmic* change in their lifestyle that Thomas did is the key to recovering from adrenal exhaustion. He needed to synchronize his life better with the Rhythms of day and night. Some people may need to allow for more down time, more leisure time, more rest, and more joy in their daily lives. It's an old saying, and it is still true: "Doing the same thing and expecting a different result is ignoring the obvious."

Healing your adrenals is not a path for the weak-willed. It takes determination to make these changes. We live in a culture that expects us to operate at a pace that would kill an elephant. The activity level at which most people function in today's fast-paced culture couldn't be more perfectly designed to deplete the adrenals.

Of course, once you've started on your program for adrenal recovery, you can motivate yourself by keeping the rewards and "punishments" in mind. Feeling better is a huge carrot, and remembering how bad you used to feel is a good stick. Two very informative books on fatigue by Dr. Jacob Teitelbaum can be extremely helpful: *From Fatigued to Fantastic*, and *The Fatigue and Fibromyalgia Solution*. And it's important to find a doctor who understands adrenal fatigue and can work with you as you journey back to vitality and aliveness.

FIBROMYALGIA

Soraya's next appointment took place about eight months from her initial visit. "I'm feeling about 80 percent back to normal," she reported cheerfully. In fact, she felt so much better that she was enthusiastic about helping others feel better, too. "My friend Bernadette has fibromyalgia," she mentioned to me. "Do you think you can help her?"

Fibromyalgia is a relatively new official medical diagnosis. However, the symptom presentation has been around for a long time, just under different guises or names. Fibromyalgia is a condition of fatigue combined with overall muscle pain. Because there is a lot of pain, it can make sleep problematic, which makes the fatigue worse. Activity is limited both because of the pain and the fatigue. It's a pretty miserable thing to experience.

I have witnessed a lot of people with fibromyalgia get better, as well as some who continue to have some pain. As with many chronic conditions, fibromyalgia can evolve from a number of different paths, all with an endpoint of some or all of the fibromyalgia symptoms. As with my process of diagnosing Soraya (and, indeed, all my patients), I have found that the key to finding the core issues is to listen carefully to the person's story. All the clues are present in the story, if I listen long enough and carefully.

"I'll do my best to find out if I can help your friend when she comes in for an appointment," I promised Soraya.

When Soraya's friend Bernadette arrived for her first appointment, I spent the first hour listening to her story, which included her present problems as well as her past health. When she felt complete, I had a lot of questions for her.

"Can you remember when the muscle pain began?" I asked, to start the process.

"Seems like it was after I had Lyme disease, about four years ago. My body never stopped hurting. I feel like I never really recovered from the Lyme," Bernadette reflected.

"How long did you take antibiotics for the Lyme disease?"

"Well, my primary-care doctor gave me three weeks of Doxycycline. When I didn't feel much better after that, I went to a Lyme doctor. She put me on a whole bunch of different antibiotics. I took them for almost a year. And I still didn't feel good!"

It was clear that Bernadette was frustrated. Still, I sensed that she hadn't lost hope of returning to wellness, or she wouldn't have come to see me. I continued, "I think your problems could be due to yeast."

The Link between Yeast (Candida) and Fibromyalgia

I pulled out the quiz for yeast (or *candida*) in Dr. William Crook's book, *The Yeast Connection and Women's Health*. Together, Bernadette and I went through the quiz and added up her score. "Your score is 15," I pointed out, "which—according to Dr. Crook—means that your health problems are almost certainly yeast-connected." (To view the "Yeast Quiz," see the Appendix at the back of this book.)

Although Bernadette was surprised, she seemed delighted that a possible cause finally had been found. "I never thought that yeast might be a problem, although I do get a lot of yeast infections. What does this mean?"

"The medical term for an overgrowth of yeast is *candidiasis*. It is an imbalance of the body's biome—the ecosystem of bacteria, viruses, and fungi that live in our body. A person with a candida overgrowth can experience many of the symptoms of fibromyalgia, such as fatigue, mental fog, muscle pain, sleep problems, and more," I explained.

I could see that Bernadette was closely following what I was saying. "Yup, that's me, all right!" she agreed.

"Unfortunately," I continued, "in medical school, doctors are taught that candidiasis only occurs in patients with suppressed immune systems—such as people with AIDS or on immunosuppressive drugs. In reality, the condition is much more widespread."

"So how did it happen to *me*?"

"Candidiasis—or *candida*, as it's commonly called—is most frequently the result of antibiotic use. Sometimes a single round of antibiotics can kill enough of our residential bacterial population that it results in a yeast overgrowth. Often, there is a repeating pattern of taking antibiotics several times a year or more for a number of years. Or an incident that resulted in taking antibiotics for several weeks or longer."

"How about taking antibiotics for almost a year?" she snorted. "Like me?"

"Sometimes," I added, "candida can result from chronic diarrhea, which washes away a lot of the normal gut bacteria and creates an imbalanced population of bacteria and yeast."

"So if candida is my problem, then if we treat the candida I could get better?" Bernadette was really excited now.

"Yes," I assured her. "In fact, I have seen it happen many times."

Treatment for candidiasis can take up to six to twelve months, and involves some dietary lifestyle changes. Avoiding simple carbohydrates and sugars needs to be a permanent change in order to maintain optimal wellness. I would recommend these same dietary guidelines for anyone seeking to maintain good health. (For a more complete explanation of candidiasis and how to treat it, please review that section in Chapter Two: "The Golden Key—Engaging the Rhythms of Good Digestion.")

"Could anything *else* be causing my fibromyalgia?" Bernadette was wondering. I imagined she was hoping for some way not to have to avoid sugar. (Sugar had featured prominently in the food diary she had brought to her appointment at my request.)

"Muscle pain *can* be caused by very low levels of Vitamin D3," I responded. "This usually resolves in a few weeks after starting adequate Vitamin D supplementation. I find that most people in temperate climates need a maintenance dose of 2,000-5,000 IU of Vitamin D3 daily. Some people need to take two or three times that much for an initial month, to rebuild their stores. Many people notice bonus effects after raising their Vitamin D3 levels. They mention that their mood improves and they have a more positive outlook on life." I could see that I still had Bernadette's full attention.

Fibromyalgia can also result from trauma. The collagen in our muscle fibers and fascia retains memory of abuse and trauma. Sometimes these memories are released unexpectedly during massage or other bodywork, and can look like shaking or tears. Some body workers are trained in how to handle these releases. I knew one physical therapist who asked her patients to bring their therapist to sessions with her so that any trauma that resurfaced would be handled with the goal of safety and healing. (To find out more about working with trauma, see Chapter Five: "The Mind-Body Connection.")

ANEMIA

Anemia can definitely cause chronic tiredness and lack of energy. The medical definition of anemia is applied when the hematocrit or hemoglobin (both reflect the number of red blood cells) fall below the range of normal. Some forms of anemia, such as iron-deficiency anemia, can also cause leg pains, cracked lips, and shortness of breath with activity. Anemia can also be the result of B12 or folate deficiencies. Or it could be a combination of all three deficiencies: iron, B12, and folate.

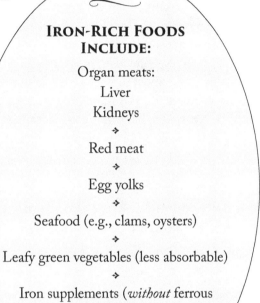

IRON-RICH FOODS INCLUDE:

Organ meats:
Liver
Kidneys
✦
Red meat
✦
Egg yolks
✦
Seafood (e.g., clams, oysters)
✦
Leafy green vegetables (less absorbable)
✦
Iron supplements (*without* ferrous sulfate)—such as:
Ferrous gluconate
Ferrous fumarate

The blood tests for checking whether you are anemic is the Complete Blood Count with differential and platelets, Vitamin B12, folate, iron and total iron-binding capacity (TIBC), and ferritin. Total iron-binding capacity is a blood test to see if you have too much or too little iron in the blood. Iron moves through the blood attached to a protein called transferrin. The TIBC test helps your doctor know how well that protein can carry iron in the blood. Ferritin is a storage form of iron. If your hemoglobin or hematocrit are below the normal range, this is the diagnosis of anemia. If your RDW is elevated, this is a sign that the body is working extra hard to make more red blood cells to correct the anemia.

It is important to determine the cause of the anemia. Once the cause of anemia has been determined, a solution can begin to be found. If the iron levels are low, it is helpful to take additional iron, both in the form of supplements and in foods. Foods that are especially rich in iron are organ meats such as liver and kidneys; red meat; egg yolks; seafood, such as clams and oysters; molasses; and prunes. Leafy green vegetables also contain iron; however, our bodies have more trouble absorbing it in this form. Studies have shown that levels of iron in spinach (Popeye's traditional energizer) have decreased to one-third of what they were fifty years ago, presumably because of the lower level of micronutrients and microflora in the soil today.

Iron supplements are easily available and come in a mind-boggling variety. The most important thing to remember is to *avoid* taking an iron supplement that contains *ferrous sulfate*. This form is typically what doctors prescribe, but it is poorly absorbed and can also cause constipation and stomach problems. Better forms of iron include ferrous gluconate or fumarate.

OTHER THINGS TO CHECK IF YOU'RE FATIGUED

If these things don't account for your symptoms of fatigue, there are still other possibilities that can be checked out.

Vitamin B12 Deficiency

Most people who come to me already have had a doctor check for anemia and have been told that they are "fine," meaning that their hematocrit and hemoglobin are within the normal range. However, not many doctors check levels of Vitamin B12 and folate. Even if these levels turn out to be normal, a level at the *low* end of the normal range may be deficient enough to cause fatigue. Another clue that either Vitamin B12 or folate may be low is the Mean Corpuscular Volume (MCV) in the CBC that is high, or higher than mid-range. Lack of either B12 or folate, or both, can result in raising the MCV, which means that the size of the red blood cells (corpuscles) are larger than average.

I once heard a talk by a doctor from Australia whose specialty was working with Vitamin B12. In his opinion, the optimal level for Vitamin B12 was 1500pg/mL. Most laboratory values have the top normal range of 900 to 1100pg/mL. Vitamin B12 is a water-soluble vitamin, and any excess that the body doesn't need is eliminated. There are no known adverse effects of having B12 levels over the normal laboratory range, so supplementation with extra B12 is relatively risk-free.

There are no known adverse effects of having B12 levels over the normal laboratory range, so supplementation with extra B12 is relatively risk-free.

If a person has low Vitamin B12 levels, several factors can be involved. The most obvious is that their B12 intake is low. Vitamin B12 is found only in animal foods, so people on a vegan diet need to supplement their diet with B12. Another cause for a B12 deficiency can be inability to *absorb* B12. Vitamin B12 has to combine with Intrinsic Factor in the stomach and then get absorbed in the terminal ileum (part of the small intestine). If a person lacks adequate stomach acid, they may not make enough Intrinsic Factor. Inadequate stomach acid is a common reason for a B12 deficiency in an older person. If they have had a gastric bypass or stomach stapling, they may no longer make adequate Intrinsic Factor or have use of their terminal ileum, and so Vitamin B12 cannot be absorbed. Parasites can also interfere with absorption of Vitamin B12.

Some Easily Absorbable Forms of Vitamin B12:

Sublingual
→
Oral sprays
→
Injections

The sublingual (melt-in-the-mouth) or oral spray form of Vitamin B12 is better absorbed, compared to swallowing a pill. If levels are not improving with a sublingual or spray supplement, then Vitamin B12 injections are helpful. I usually start with weekly intramuscular injections of 1000 mcg of the methylcobalamin form of B12. Some people need to take it more frequently. After a month or two, the interval between injections can be extended, as tolerated. Some people begin to be able to absorb oral Vitamin B12 much better after getting shots for a while.

Folic–Acid Deficiency

Sometimes the MCV is higher than mid-range because of a folate (folic acid) deficiency. Folate deficiencies are less common than Vitamin B12 deficiencies, and can be remedied with sublingual or oral folic acid supplements. If the MCV is high, it is important to supplement not just folate but also Vitamin B12. While replacing only folate can result in an improvement in the MCV, this can mask an underlying Vitamin B12 deficiency.

MTHFR-INDUCED FATIGUE

Methylenetetrahydrofolate reductase (MTHFR) is the rate-limiting enzyme in the methyl cycle. The *MTHFR* gene provides instructions for making the enzyme called methylenetetrahydrofolate reductase. This enzyme plays a role in processing amino acids, the building blocks of proteins. Methylenetetrahydrofolate reductase is important for a chemical reaction involving forms of the vitamin folate, also called Vitamin B9. Specifically, this enzyme converts a molecule called 5,10-methylenetetrahydrofolate to a molecule called 5-methyltetrahydrofolate. This reaction is required for the multi-step process that converts the amino acid homocysteine to another amino acid, methionine.

The body uses methionine to make proteins and other important compounds. Methylation is an important biochemical process, vital to a large number of biochemical pathways involving neurotransmitters, detoxification, cardiovascular health, eye health, muscle health, bone health, and redox balance.

Several variations in the MTHFR gene (also known as polymorphisms) have been associated with an increased risk of neural-tube defects. Some mutations in this gene are associated with methylenetetrahydrofolate reductase deficiency. Dysfunction of the methylation process is thought to possibly have additional effects, and investigations are ongoing.

There has been recent interest in testing for the MTHFR gene to see whether someone is heterozygous or homozygous for a deficiency of this gene. Someone who is *homozygous* is deficient in both genes that code for the enzyme, which may significantly impair their ability to methylate.

Someone who is *heterozygous* may have some impairment but not, it is thought, as significantly.

I have tested some people for the MTHFR gene, particularly those who seem to have difficulty returning to a state of good health after an illness such as Lyme or Epstein-Barr. These people often say they never felt well since they had a particular bout of illness. If the tests show that they are homozygous for MTHFR, it seems to help to supplement with methylated folate, methylated Vitamin B12 and Vitamin B6, and activated riboflavin. Some people have noticed an improvement in their sense of wellbeing when taking these supplements.

This was the advice I gave to Bernadette.

"I think I get it!" Bernadette nodded. "You're helping me rule out everything that might be working against me, and undertake a lifestyle that will make me well and strong again. I'm tired of being tired—and thanks to our collaboration, I believe I can look forward to feeling energetic. And I am willing to do whatever I need to do."

"Thank you, Bernadette," I said warmly. "You are not only a good patient, you're also a good self-healer! At this point, you have a wonderful prognosis, and I look forward to working with you."

Emotional Health and Chronic Fatigue

Our emotional health is another key to recovering vitality and good health.

Rebecca is a patient I see and talk to often, because she seems to get sick a lot. She will call or come in, and I usually review the list of vitamins and herbs that will help her recover from the current cold or sinus problem that seems to plague her. At her last visit in the office, I noticed how wan and listless she seemed.

Since I felt that we had developed sufficient trust between us over time, I undertook to delve a little deeper. I asked her, "Tell me a little more about your life. What is your typical day and week like?"

"Well," she sighed, "I have my job, which is very stressful. There are always deadlines, and I never know if the job will end at any time. And when I'm not working, I go over to help take care of my mother. I think I'm depressed. Actually, I've been depressed for years."

"Do you enjoy your work?"

"No, I hate it. But I only have three years until I retire, so I'm hanging in." Her voice was flat and devoid of any enthusiasm.

"And what will you do when you retire?"

"I guess then I will just take care of my mother," she responded in the same lackluster tone.

We sat in silence, contemplating her future as she had painted it. Finally I said, "It feels to me like you are living in shoes too small for you. What is needed is a bigger vision for yourself, so that your life becomes an adventure rather than a test of endurance."

I paused to see her reaction. I was a little worried that maybe I was pushing a little too hard, and yet I could sense her feeling lost and despondent.

After a moment her eyes lit up. "That's exactly right!" she exclaimed. "I need a bigger vision. That's what I want!" She was looking much more alive and present, now. "But how do I begin?"

I suggested, "Perhaps a good place to start might be to look at the fears that are blocking you from stepping into a bigger vision for your life. Maybe make a list of the fears. See if those fears are based on your current reality, or are they perhaps fears that you picked up from your family when you were young and later took on as your own. You could evaluate whether your fears are running the show, and consider how things might be different if they weren't."

Rebecca left looking much more alive than when she had arrived. And *I* also felt more alive. What I had said to her, I needed to hear as well. I know that the challenge of looking at our fears is no small undertaking. Neither is taking a risk and opening to new possibilities. But when our life feels joyless, an endless rote performance of routines, we have lost our vitality. Sickness and depression can be ways to stay numb. We are *surviving*, but not *thriving*. We have lost sight of the gift of *being* in a human body, *fully alive* in our life.

Some Final Words on Fatigue and Recovery

Chronic fatigue is a signal from our body that our energy is low, as well as a signal from our emotions that we are not experiencing joy in life. Take a good look at how you dance with the Rhythms of *work and play*, and *rest and activity*.

Are you surviving but not *thriving*? If your life seems like "wearing a tight shoe," look into what living a larger life might involve. Enlist the help and support of a knowledgeable mentor or practitioner. Explore all the possible factors contributing to your fatigue. All this is part of rebalancing and harmonizing with Life's Rhythms —the key to full recovery of vitality.

CHAPTER TEN

OPTIMAL AGEING: THE CROWN OF LIFE

The Rhythm of Generosity and Reciprocity

"I choose to make the rest of my life the best of my life."   —Louise Hay

"The afternoon knows what the morning never suspected."
—Robert Frost

The Rhythms of Life flow through us. We are each a tiny wave on the ocean, and eventually our wave will crash on the beach and be no more. Ageing is like watching the ebb tide. Until it happens to us, we think getting old is something that happens only to other people. I remember once talking with my mother-in-law, a very wise woman and close to ninety at the time. She said, "The funny thing is I still feel the same inside—like that young girl I used to be."

When Do We Start to Notice That We Are Ageing?

Maybe it's in our late thirties or early forties, when we notice that we can't quite keep up with the kids like we used to. Or when achy joints and stiffness in the morning become noticeable. Or when our night vision isn't as good as it used to be, or we need to use reading glasses. Or our hair begins to thin and gray. Maybe we didn't really take notice until our fifties or sixties. We had ourselves convinced that, really, ageing was just somehow going to bypass us. We lived in denial of the Universal Rhythms of Birth and Death, Growth and Decay.

Whatever the specific wakeup call we get, eventually we come to the point where we acknowledge that we are ageing and that, despite all our best efforts, some changes are happening. Perhaps if we lived in a culture that *valued* the old ones, we would not be so resistant to ageing. We might perhaps experience less fear and anxiety and have a more gracious acceptance and perhaps, even joy. What if our society had a real appreciation for elder wisdom and revered the old ones as treasures of the community?

ARE YOU BECOMING AN *ELDER*, OR JUST OLDER?

All of us are getting older. No choice there. However, some of us will perhaps choose to become an *elder*. An elder is one who has climbed to the crown of the tree of knowledge. At the crown or top of the tree, one has the biggest horizon, the widest view. From this highest place we have a different perspective about our life than when we were down in the lower branches. At the top of the tree, things that were obscured by leaves and branches lower down are now seen more clearly. *This broader vision is at the core of elder wisdom.* We see the people, values, and issues in our life within a larger perspective, and can make wiser choices on that basis.

Grandchildren can give one a sense of roots, a deepening sense of our place in the generational tree. We can also attain this sense of rootedness from a garden we have long cared for, or another beloved long-term project. Each time we enter our "garden," we note new developments and changes, just as one might note in a grandchild seen over time. As elders, we begin to understand the Native American teaching that important decisions should be made using the wisdom of the previous seven generations and with the perspective of their effect on the next seven generations.

Being an Elder

Elders have learned to modulate the sense of urgency and rush that permeates our culture. Our pace slows and becomes more measured. We give greater value to the savoring of the moment, finding joy in what we have been given, and we appreciate the ability of laughter to lighten the load. We value our authenticity and listen for our inner truth rather than socially accepted expectations.

Our world *needs* elders. Many women hunger for mentoring from a woman elder. Many men yearn for an elder man's approval and guidance. It is human nature to seek out teachers and mentors to help guide us through life's journeys. These are the greatest gifts that an elder has to offer—the gift of guidance, and especially the gift of blessing.

An elder has gleaned wisdom from sifting through a lifetime of experiences. Elders no longer fear the repercussions of speaking their truth. There is a sense that life is too short to mince words or avoid taking a stand. In our world, the greatest truth speakers are the very young and the very old. One speaks from the place of innocence, and the other from the place of wisdom.

In the elder phase of life, it is important to take time to review your life journey and harvest the wisdom you have gained. Are there ways in which you may be hiding from assuming your duties as an elder? Are there younger people hungry for mentoring whom you are ignoring? Perhaps you have gotten a little stuck in your comfort zone and need to stretch into elderhood? Opportunities abound for an elder to give back to family and to community. Rather than accept our society's current de-valuing of old people, "Be the change you want to see in the world," as Gandhi said.

On Mentors and Mentoring

One of the greatest gifts we can give ourselves is to find a mentor or mentors to help guide us. The gift of guidance is rare and precious, both for the mentor and the mentee. I feel very fortunate to have been mentored by some exceptional teachers.

I personally use a "Board of Advisors" as a tool for guidance to help me sort through the many realms in my life. When I am unclear or uninformed and feel the need for help, I seek out the appropriate Board member. I chose one who is particularly skillful in finances, another whose parenting approach I admire greatly, yet another whose way of holding spiritual growth and work I wish to emulate, and another whose creativity is inspirational. Some of these people are my friends, some are my teachers, and some are generous colleagues. As I become aware of a new realm that I wish to master, I look for support and advice from someone who already has mastery in that realm.

As we age, we get opportunities to mentor others in turn, sharing the wisdom we have gained. In doing this, we dance with the Rhythms of Reciprocity and Generosity.

> *As elders, when we mentor others and share the wisdom we have gained, we dance with the Rhythms of reciprocity and generosity.*

Physical Changes of Ageing

My father used to say, "Growing old is like watching the cookie crumble." As we age, our bodies lose muscle tone, our skin begins to sag and wrinkle and strange spots and bumps develop. We need glasses to read, and we no longer take the stairs two at a time. We may tire more easily, or experience stiffness when we rise in the morning or after being still. If we over-used or abused our bodies when we were younger, we now reap the consequences in additional pain and disabilities or other difficulties. Our digestion or sleep may become problematic. Memory, especially new learning, becomes more difficult.

It is important to re-evaluate our medications as we age. The older body can be more sensitive to medications and their complex interactions. I have met many older adults who are taking a number of different medications, some that they started years ago. A blood-pressure medicine that was helpful when you were forty or fifty and dealing with a highly stressful job as well as many other stresses may no longer be necessary in old age. A common side effect of too much blood-pressure medication is lightheadedness, which can cause missteps and falls. Cholesterol-lowering medicine can impede Vitamin D absorption, which is important for bone health. Acid-blocking medicine can reduce protein digestion and uptake of minerals.

I remind my older patients that caring for an older body is like caring for an older car. Expect to spend more, both in terms of time and money, on maintenance and upkeep. Think of this older body as a priceless heirloom that you have inherited and want to keep in the best condition possible.

*Think of your older body as a priceless heirloom
that you have inherited and want to keep in the
best condition possible.*

The Need for Touch

We humans enjoy physical touch. We are *sensual* and *sexual* creatures. To look at ourselves and disregard this is pure folly. We know that touch is vital in order for human beings to continue to thrive. Babies who do not get held or touched develop "failure to thrive," and some even die as a result.

Richard Horton, editor-in-chief of the science journal *The Lancet*, wrote: "The avoidance of touch is bad medicine.... Touch builds trust, reassurance and a sense of communion." And novelist Margaret Atwood wrote in *The Blind Assassin*, "Touch comes before sight, before speech. It is the first language and the last, and it always tells the truth."

It has been said that human beings need *a minimum of four hugs a day to survive* and *more to thrive.* Many of us are not really getting enough touch on a daily basis to thrive. If this inspires you to go out and get more hugs on a daily basis, good! However, I have some advice: rather than assume that people will want to hug, before approaching them with your arms spread wide ask them, "Are you available for a hug?" Sometimes people may *not* be available at that moment. They will appreciate your consideration. And chances are you will get a lot more real hugs than if you had never asked.

I have a dog that comes over for some touch when she starts to feel anxious. Her nose will nudge me, and when I pet her she rolls over on her back and wants me to rub her tummy. We are *all* sensual creatures. Positive physical contact, loving touch, is essential to our wellbeing. Without it we simply don't thrive. Hugs and touch create *the Rhythm of Generosity and Reciprocity*—as we give, we also receive at the same time.

Sex and Ageing

As we age, our sex drive usually wanes. The biological drive to make babies is gone. Hormone levels of estrogen and testosterone start to decline by age forty. Many women tell me of their distress that they no longer have the same interest and desire for sex as they did when they were younger. Men also note a decline in the intensity of their sexual desire. Erectile function decreases due to decreased testosterone levels, and to reduced elasticity in blood vessels through ageing, diabetes, or atherosclerosis. Women need more time to become fully aroused, and many menopausal women note decreased lubrication and pain with intercourse.

If you want to continue to be sexually active in your elder years, using bio-identical hormones can be helpful. These hormones can help with vaginal lubrication and elasticity, as well as libido and erectile function. However, it is important to have your hormone levels checked both *before* and *while* taking hormone replacement, to make sure that you stay in the physiological normal range.

Bio-identical hormones are made by compounding pharmacies. These hormones are identical to the hormones the human body makes but are synthesized in a laboratory. Check with your local compounding pharmacies to get names of doctors who prescribe them if you don't know of any. (For more information on bio-identical hormones, see Chapter Seven: Menopause.)

DEATH AND DYING

Elders walk with death perched like a raven on their shoulder. They know that the death door lies ahead. Living with the raven, each day becomes a precious gift to be appreciated.

My question is: are we ready for our death?

"Why Do I Have Such a Hard Time Accepting That I Will Die?"

The truth is, we know it's coming. Sooner or later, that black-cloaked figure with the scythe will knock on our door. The signs are there. The skin is starting to look like crepe paper. Bags under the eyes don't disappear, even after a good night's sleep. There's the slow creep of wither and shrink. Yet in the hustle and bustle of life, it is hard to stay mindful of the raven perched on our shoulder and to keep that perspective.

What is this life that we are given supposed to be *about*? We continue to build on some belief or other—success, love, children, creativity, our plans, dreams. Are these just stories we tell ourselves? One thing dies, and then another. We watch Mother Nature each year as she takes down her creation and lets it die. We watch it shrivel and fade, lose color and form, and ultimately become grey skeletons turning into compost and returning back to the earth.

Frantically, we attempt to hold back the tide with creams and potions, hair dyes, regimens of exercise and diet, even surgery—alas, ultimately all for naught. As the tide came in, so the tide will inevitably go out. Death, the Grim Reaper, will finally find us, each and every one of us, with no exception.

Is there anything to be done? Is a "bucket list" important? Is *any* list important, given the enormity of Death looming ahead? The words not spoken, the deeds not done, the quilt unsewn, the song unsung?

Has it been enough? Is it *ever* enough? Do we ever know when we've had enough, or it is just a matter of living becoming too much trouble to endure any more? Some say, "Death is like taking off a tight shoe." Many of us have difficulty believing that one day, we will be no more.

How to Prepare for Death

We get our house in order.

Many older people have spoken to me about feeling a need to clear out the clutter in their homes and lives. They have begun to disperse their possessions, to lighten up their burden of material goods and responsibilities. For many, it seems that a sense of urgency develops in the sixties. We want to clean up while we still have the faculties and strength to do it. And there is something very vitalizing in letting go of all that stuff!

One of my patients and her husband chose to sell their home after retiring. They put a few chosen possessions into storage and took off to travel around the country in a small RV. They took two years, visiting places they had always wanted to explore. When my patient returned for an appointment two years later, she seemed revitalized, energized, and greatly satisfied with her and her spouse's decision to release their moorings and follow their dreams. Other older patients have chosen to downsize to a small home or apartment, or have moved in with adult children and their families. They, too, seem to find their new chosen life more stimulating and rewarding.

The key to graceful ageing seems to begin with a fierce and truthful acceptance of our situation—the physical, financial, and emotional limitations and assets—and finding the best solution for ourselves. No one can know what will happen in the future, so we make the best decision we can, based on what we know now. This is an act of great courage. Facing our fears and opening to change—these are heroic acts.

How Do We Live Our Lives Fully Unto Death?

Sometimes when I sit with my older patients, I ask if they have thought about their death and how they want it to be and not to be.

It's not an easy subject to discuss for many people. Most of us would rather not think about it, thank you very much. *But now here's Dr. Rothschild asking me all these questions, and I am forced to look at it. Do I want to die at home? Do I want heroic measures to be taken if my heart should stop or my breathing cease? Have I thought about designing my funeral? Gee, Dr. Rothschild, that's a lot to think about!*

An old friend of mine, Paul, was diagnosed with cancer and knew that he was going to die in less than a year. He chose to spend the time he had left visiting all his friends in various parts of the country to say goodbye. He was widely known and well loved by many people who had worked with him in community-service programs in several states over the years. In one town, a group of his friends organized a memorial service for him, to which he was invited to be the guest of honor. It was a most extraordinarily moving experience for everyone present—including Paul. Not many people get to attend their own memorial service and hear the tributes and stories that their loved ones speak from their hearts. Paul was a man who allowed himself to live his life fully—even into his death.

Another amazing story about dying involves a friend of mine, Allan. Allan came from a very close-knit family that was decidedly undemonstrative. There was deep love between them, but the words "I love you" were never spoken, and displays of physical affection were rare. Allan had been a musician and a teacher, and also had served as choir director at his church for many years. As he lay on his deathbed, his whole family—including his children and all the grandchildren—gathered around him.

He had been very quiet that day. Suddenly he sat up in bed and, looking around at them all, he began to sing, "I love you, I love you, I love you" over and over and over. Then he lay back down.

Forty-five minutes later, surrounded by family, he stopped breathing.

Living Wills and Last Words

It's never too late to have the last word, until it *is* too late and we are dead. And, as I said earlier, it is helpful to plan how we want to die. Dr. Kevorkian gave this country the gift of conscious death. We *can* make some choices around dying before we die.

Personally, I know that I do not want to die a slow death, dwindling over the years and losing my faculties bit by bit. Nor do I relish the idea of being a burden on my children. I have always said that I will keep a bottle of pills on the mantelpiece with the injunction, "If you can't remember what these are for, TAKE THEM!" I'm only half-joking.

My preferences for dying are in this order: first, to die in my sleep; second, to die from a massive heart attack or stroke; or third, to discover that I have cancer and die a week later, like my old friend, Martha. I definitely do *not* want to be resuscitated in the event that my heart stops or I stop breathing. My wish is to have no life-saving interventions, and I have made sure that my children know my wishes.

Today, many people are aware of Living Wills. A Living Will is basically a written statement of your personal preferences regarding emergency medical treatment in the event that you are unconscious, your heart or breathing stops, or you are in a condition that renders you unable to communicate. Many such forms can be found online, and most hospitals also have these forms. Take some time to make your Living Will; then tell those who need to know what you want, or give them a copy.

When I was a medical resident working in a hospital, one of my duties was to interview and examine each patient when he or she was first admitted into the hospital. Part of that interview included discussing whether the patient wished to be designated "Do Not Resuscitate" (DNR) or not. I had to inquire if this newly admitted patient had thought about what she or he wanted to be done, should their heart stop beating or their breathing stop. In other words, I had to initiate a discussion with the patient about their death and how they wanted to die.

It was not an easy subject for me to bring up, and most people were uncomfortable and unprepared to talk about it. Yet I had to do it. It didn't matter whether they came in to have a hernia repair or brain surgery. The hospital wanted to be sure that it was following the patient's wishes. My responsibility was to note in their chart whether or not the patient wanted extraordinary measures to be taken, such as CPR and electroshock and intubation with artificial respiration. After my interview, those new patients' wishes were then clearly documented in their chart. If they did not want any interventions, a big orange sticker labeled "DNR" was put on their chart so that no one could miss it and mistakenly start resuscitation.

We don't talk much about death in our culture. It's taboo. We feel ill at ease or awkward with the subject. Doctors are no different. Many are uncomfortable with death, themselves, and avoid bringing the subject up with their patients.

Even though many of the patients I interviewed in the hospital were seriously ill, embarking on a conversation about death and dying often seemed to come as a complete shock to them. For my part, I found that it required a certain amount of courage and delicacy to bring up the topic with these people whom I had just met. Sometimes I had the sense that they had never given their own death a thought, prior to my question. With others, it was clear that they had thought it over and knew exactly what they wanted. The most surprising thing I discovered was that many patients were *relieved* to be asked. They *wanted* their wishes known. They had thought about their death, and they had clear preferences. The hardest part was just broaching the topic of death.

Clarence was one of the many patients I admitted as a resident. During that hospital stay, he was diagnosed with pancreatic cancer. When we first met, Clarence was a big man—strong, physically active, and in the prime of his life. Looking at him, it was hard to believe that he had cancer.

Six months later, I found myself in the Intensive Care Unit (ICU) of the hospital one night. Looking over the charts, I noticed that Clarence was in one of the ICU rooms. When I went in to see him, I found his physical appearance to be a shock. He had shrunk to a shell of his former robust self. There were four tubes running fluids into him and four lines carrying fluids out. As I read the various notes that his doctors had put in his chart, I learned that he had undergone many procedures in the previous months, and still more were planned.

However, there was no mention in the notes of whether he had been asked as to his wishes regarding death and artificial resuscitation. The nurses confirmed that his doctors had not broached the subject with him. (The hospital did not allow the *nurses* to initiate that conversation.)

It was late, but Clarence was awake. I approached his bed and introduced myself, and he remembered me. We talked a little; and then I mentioned, in a gentle way, that things did not look very hopeful and he agreed. I asked him how he felt about dying, and he said that he was ready. I asked if he had told his wife and son that he was ready. He replied that he had not. I asked if he would like me to call them to come in so that he could talk with them and tell them. He said he would. I went to the nurses' station and called his wife and son, and asked if they could come in, as he wanted to talk with them. They arrived within the hour and sat with him.

It was such a sacred moment. Tears and much love were expressed. With the nurse and I standing by as witnesses, Clarence said that he did not wish to have further life-saving measures taken. He told his family that he was ready to die, and that he loved them and was sorry to leave them. They told him how much they loved him, and that they didn't want him to suffer any more. They reassured him that they would be all right and that they were ready to let him go. After some time together, including many tears and hugs, they left.

With the nurse as my witness, I put the "Do Not Resuscitate" order on Clarence's chart. Very late that same night, he passed away.

Getting Ready for Death

"Plant your garden for your children's children, and enjoy your garden as if this is your last day on earth."　　　　　　　　　　—Anonymous

We can at least make a plan for the end and let our loved ones know how we feel about our death. We can put our finances and physical possessions in order, to make the passing of the baton as easeful as possible for those who will have to take it up next.

There are many wonderful and amazing stories of people's end-of-life experiences. Stephen and Ondrea Levine ran a hotline for five years for people who were "sitting bedside" with people as they were dying. Over the years they heard some amazing stories, which they put into a book titled *Meetings at the Edge*. And Elizabeth Kubler-Ross, a Swiss physician, was a pioneer in removing the taboo about talking about death. Her work in the 1960s included many books on death and dying, including one especially written for children called *Remember the Secret.* Another book that helps us focus our intentions around dying is *With the End in Mind* by Kathryn Mannix. It is full of insights and wisdom gleaned from years of working with people at the end of life as a palliative-care physician.

My own experiences of being with people who are dying seem very similar to what I felt as a midwife being around births. It is the same Miracle of Life being witnessed. With one, the door swings into Life; with the other the door swings out of Life into Death. I feel very honored to be present at these times, to witness the amazing miracle and mystery that is Life.

At birth, when a baby's body emerges it begins to glow as Life moves into it—truly a miracle. Sometimes babies are born grey and floppy, and need to be rubbed and talked to and urged to join the living before they pink up and enter Life. And I have seen a baby born grey and still who never took a breath, and it was clear and palpable that there was no Life present in that baby's body.

I have experienced this same sense of awe and awareness of the simultaneous presence of "life" and "no life" when sitting at a deathbed. There is a palpable difference between the presence of Life in a dying person and the lack of that presence after they die. Even though they may be very weak or even unconscious, there is a sense that something is still there in that body. Once that intangible something leaves the body, the body becomes like a shell. It may bear a resemblance to the person we knew and loved, but the intrinsic quality that was the spark of that person is gone. The miracle of Life has exited that body and is present no more. It is important to honor this passing and take as much care in planning the exit as one takes in planning the entrance of a baby.

Give yourself permission to muse on your own death and possible scenarios. Pick your favorite options. Of course, you may not get your first choice—or your second, for that matter. But giving the matter some thought decreases the fear factor and allows greater ease to flow around our inevitable farewell. And if you do or do not wish to be resuscitated, inform those close to you as well as your doctor. Consider getting a bracelet or medallion to wear that clearly states "DNR."

CANCER

It is impossible to talk about death without talking about cancer. For most people, being given the diagnosis of cancer is tantamount to being given a calling card from the Grim Reaper himself with the inscription, "I am waiting for you." Cancer, like death, is greatly feared in our culture. Yet in today's world, cancer is widespread and many of us will have a chance to dance with the options after being diagnosed with cancer.

My lovely neighbor Martha lived on the farm down the road from me. Over the years, she taught me many things, including how to make souse and dandelion wine. When I met her, she was in her seventies. A small, energetic woman, she had birthed twelve children, and each Sunday she hosted dinner for her entire clan. Her kitchen had two stoves and two refrigerators, and her dining room was one long table from end to end. She still kept chickens, sold eggs, and mowed her own lawn with a push mower in her short shorts. She was active and lively—until one day, she felt stomach pain and went to the hospital. A week later, she was dead of pancreatic cancer.

Over the years, I have met many people who have had cancer. Some arrived at my door already having been given the diagnosis. With others, we made the journey of discovery together. Some chose to follow their oncologist's suggestions to the letter. Others chose only to make changes in diet and lifestyle. Some spent time and money traveling to clinics and hospitals around the world dedicated to treating cancer with alternative methods not available in the United States. Still others chose combinations of the above. And others chose to continue their lives and to change nothing. Some died quite soon after being diagnosed; others lived for many years; and some are still living and doing well.

In my role as physician-guide with my patients, I have always found that trusting my patient's own knowing proves best. My role is often to lay out the options that I am aware of, and then to encourage the patients to take time to explore the direction that they feel most drawn toward. Ultimately, I recommend that they follow their inner guidance. There are no wrong or right choices. No one can predict the future. No one can guarantee that one approach will be more successful than another. Death lies at the end of the road for all of us. Our only choice is how we live in the "now" until that moment of our death.

When I consult with my patients with cancer, we meet along with their significant others. Together, we review what the tests might mean, what the options entail, how their decisions might impact their families and all else that is going on in their lives. Many feel pressured by well-meaning doctors, as well as by family and friends. We talk about those pressures. I am there with them—to support, educate, and, above all, to listen. My goal is to help them sort through the myriad facts, myths, and possibilities, and to find their own way through the choices. Each person's way is unique and uniquely right for them. I encourage them to take their time, to detach themselves as much as possible from the pressures, and to avoid making choices from a place of fear. Good decisions rarely come out of fear or haste.

Rose came to me with a large tumor in her breast. It was about the size of a tennis ball. She must have known about it for quite a while before seeking my advice. After examining the lump, we spent time talking over her options. She decided to get a biopsy to confirm that it was cancer. It was.

Rose was clear: "I do not want to have surgery, nor any chemotherapy or radiation." She told me, "I want my life to continue as it has been." She was a highly talented painter and devoted her time to her art, her family, and her garden. She chose to eat a clean diet, adding in carrot juice. And when I saw her next, she said, "I feel really well, in fact, better than I have in years!" She and her husband drew very close, and their love deepened more than ever before. She also traveled and spent time with her sister and mother, who lived far away.

A year-and-a-half later, Rose called me. "I suddenly feel weak and uncomfortable," she said. After some discussion and a house call, hospice was called in and palliative measures were taken to assure her comfort. Two weeks later, she died quietly and peacefully in her own bed, with her husband at her side. At her funeral, her husband and other family members approached me, thanking me for supporting her in her choices regarding her cancer. They, too, had noted and honored the graceful way she had fully flowered during her last years.

"Can I Go Against My Oncologist's Recommendations?"

When dealing with a cancer diagnosis, few doctors are trained to offer their patients the equally viable option of making *quality* of life the highest priority rather than *quantity* of life. The only options they typically offer are choices between various aggressive procedures such as surgery, radiation, or chemotherapy. These may have painful and debilitating effects, decreasing the quality of life and producing only small benefits in prolonging the quantity of life.

You cannot go to a man selling oranges and expect to find apples. A surgeon will offer surgery, an oncologist will know of a clinical trial with an experimental drug, and a radiation oncologist will suggest radiation. In truth, the number of deaths from cancer, with few exceptions, has not changed much despite all the new technology.

No doctor wants to destroy your hope. However, perhaps the key is to *refine your hope*. Immortality is not an option. One can choose, however, to hope for a life that feels fulfilled and complete at the end.

"How Can I Help a Dear Friend Who Has Cancer?"

In his book *Being Mortal*, Dr. Atul Gawande discusses what he learned from a palliative-care specialist, Susan Block. According to her, the most important thing that is needed by patients with a terminal diagnosis is support in dealing with their overwhelming anxiety—about death, about suffering, about loved ones and finances. She explains that it takes time to arrive at an acceptance of one's mortality and obtain a clear understanding about the promise and limits of medicine.

If you want to support your friend with a terminal diagnosis, there are some important rules to observe, according to Susan Block. Take time; do as much listening as talking. *You are helping them determine what is most important to them under the circumstances*—not which treatment option to choose. There are certain ways to speak that can be helpful to bring clarity. The words you choose make a difference. These questions involve what I call a "fierce conversation."

Some key points suggested by Susan Block include:

- Don't ask, "What do you want when you are dying?" Instead, ask, "If time becomes short, what is most important to you?" Before any decisions are made, clarity is needed.

- Ask:

  "What do you understand your prognosis to be?"

"What are your concerns about what lies ahead?"

"What kind of trade-offs are you willing to make?"

"How do you want to spend your time, if your health worsens?"

"Who do you want to make decisions for you if you become unable to respond?"

Taking the time to clarify these values allows people who are facing a terminal illness to greatly reduce anxiety. It facilitates them to take back the reins of their life and create the life they want in the time that is left.

> *Taking the time to clarify these values allows people who are facing a terminal illness to greatly reduce anxiety.*

For those of us who haven't yet realized that Life is itself a terminal diagnosis, we could benefit by having the same fierce conversation with ourselves: "What is most important to me? How do I want to spend my remaining time? What trade-offs am I willing to make? Who do I want to make decisions for me if I can't?"

The process of coming to the answers that feel right will take time and reflection. It will also serve to relieve anxiety and make what time is left more satisfying and peaceful.

"HOW CAN I STAY AS HEALTHY AS POSSIBLE AS I AGE?"

Here it is in a nutshell:

- *Make sure your digestion is working well.*
- *Get plenty of fresh air and exercise.*
- *Avoid unnecessary medical procedures and medications.*
- *Stay out of hospitals.*
- *Keep learning new things.*
- *Remember to dance with and enjoy the Rhythms of Life!*

Epilogue

I am often asked by my patients how they can find a doctor "like me" for their sister or mother or cousin or friend who lives in another part of the country. Partnering with a holistic health practitioner can be quite helpful for someone on a healing journey.

There are many resources that can assist in the search. Lists of physicians with holistic training can be found through the American Board of Integrative and Holistic Medicine, and the Institute for Functional Medicine. One can also check listings of doctors trained in Naturopathy, Orthomolecular Medicine, Homeopathy, Ayurveda, and Oriental Medicine. (Some holistic medical organizations and their contact information are included in the Appendix under the "Epilogue" section).

WHAT TO LOOK FOR IN A HOLISTIC MEDICAL PRACTITIONER

Titles and degrees alone do not guarantee the qualities of a good partner for you. I would suggest that you look for a practitioner who practices these principles:

- **Meets you eye-to-eye:** Takes enough time to sit down and hear your whole story. Acknowledges, respects, and understands your concerns.

- **Touches where it hurts:** Is not afraid to touch you, to examine you carefully, and to fully assess your condition, situation, needs, and wishes.

- **Uses the "Tincture of Time":** Sometimes, we need to wait because a problem or situation needs more time before what is really going on becomes clear.

- **Always considers the equally viable option of doing nothing when considering options for treatment:** "Doing nothing" can mean giving things concerning your wellbeing more time to reveal themselves, or allowing time to think through the various possible scenarios, or taking time to do further investigation. It can also mean taking time for a well-needed break from focusing on the problem and stepping back to obtain a new perspective. Sometimes, choosing to wait rather than rushing into action is a wiser and safer option.

- Is not afraid to say, "I don't know the answer," and also says, "I'll help you find more information": Commits to partnering with you on your health journey.

These are gems of advice I received from my own mentors, and they have guided me well over the years.

REMEMBER TO RELY ON YOURSELF

And to the above considerations, I would add one more for *you* to practice:

- **Trust your own Knowing:** *No one knows your body and what is going on in it better than you.* The key to attaining and maintaining health lies in learning to be aware of, to listen to, and to trust the messages you get from within yourself. Some of us have bodies that are like a Stradivarius; others are like bass drums. We are each unique, and your health partner should trust that *you* are your own ultimate expert.

FINDING THE RIGHT PRACTITIONER FOR YOU

How do you determine which doctors or practitioners have the desired qualities?

Consider calling their office to see if you can schedule a five- or ten-minute phone call. You want a practitioner who *wants* to meet you halfway. The kind who is aware of the importance of being able to work together as much as you are. They will be putting *you* through a screening (during the phone call) as much as you will be doing with *them*.

For example, my office assistant, who has worked with me for over ten years, is very helpful when people call with inquiries about my practice. When she can't answer their queries directly, she passes their information on to me and I give them a call. Often, I can tell after just a brief conversation whether I might be helpful and a good fit for a prospective patient. Sometimes, I can tell that a prospective patient's concern isn't in my area of expertise, and I will suggest someone else for the person to contact. I might as well tell them up front and save them time and money. On your part, if there is a good fit between you and the doctor you're interviewing, you'll know it.

Another way to learn more about a practitioner is to ask for names of some of their patients whom you could talk to (after getting the patients' permission first, of course). The Internet is another resource for viewing patients' comments about a practitioner whom you are researching.

BEGIN AT THE BEGINNING

Take responsibility for your own health by sharpening your skills of observation and self-knowledge. Know that you are the key expert for what is going on in your body. Make a plan for one first step.

Remember—*all journeys begin with the first step.*

I wish you well on your journey of health and vitality. May you dance with the Rhythms of Life!

Appendix

CHAPTER ONE—SYNCHRONY: DANCING WITH THE UNIVERSAL RHYTHMS OF LIFE

The Universal Laws

The medical intuitive Carolyn Myss says that the Universal Laws (or Laws of the Universe) reflect how creation works around us and within us. They are the laws of creation, and everything is subject to them. According to Myss, these Laws of the Universe *are* the nature of God. Here is her delineation of these universal principles, according to my interpretation:

1. **Action and reaction**—For every action, there is a reaction.
2. **The law of vibration**—All life vibrates. Everything you say, think, or do sends vibrational patterns into motion. Everything you do matters.
3. **Cause and effect**—Magnetic attraction.
4. **The law of sensation**—Your heart has the capacity to sense the hearts of all life. We are attuned to all of life.
5. **Energy comes before matter.**
6. **All life is interconnected.**
7. **The law of gravitas**—What we assign gravitas to incarnates. How choice becomes matter.

The Lunar Calendar

The Lunar Calendar is available through:
Luna Press
P. O. Box 15511
Kenmore Station
Boston, MA 02215-0009
(617) 327-8000
www.thelunapress.com

Books

Ebun Laughing Crow Adelona, Ph.D. *Save Yourself: A Practical Guide for Understanding Energy, Emotions and Health*. Hot Springs, South Dakota: Audver Books, 2002.

Pema Chodron. *When Things Fall Apart: Heart Advice for Difficult Times.* Boston and London: Shambhala Publications, 1996.

James Hollis, Ph.D. *Swamplands of the Soul: New Life in Dismal Places.* Toronto, Canada: Inner City Books, 1996.

Carolyn Myss. *Anatomy of the Spirit: The Seven Stages of Healing.* Cuba, MO: Three Rivers Press, 1996.

_____. *Energy Anatomy.* Louisville, CO: Sounds True, 1997.

CHAPTER TWO—THE GOLDEN KEY: ENGAGING THE RHYTHMS OF GOOD DIGESTION

Lab Tests

Here are some labs that test for Leaky Gut, gut flora, parasites, and yeast overgrowth:

Doctor's Data, Inc.
3755 Illinois Avenue
St. Charles, IL 60174-2420
Phone: 1-800-323-2784
E-mail: *info@doctorsdata.com*
Website: *www.doctorsdata.com*

Genova Diagnostics
63 Zukkucia Street
Asheville, NC 28801
Phone: 1-800-522-4762
Website: *www.gdx.net*

Great Plains Laboratory, Inc.
11813 West 77th Street
Lenexa, KS 66214
Phone: 1-800-288-0383
E-mail: *customerservice@gpl4u.com*
Website: *www.greatplainslaboratory.com*

Food Allergies

The Allergy Elimination Diet
Reprinted with permission from Alan R. Gaby, M.D., *Nutritional Medicine*, 2nd Edition. Concord, NH: Fritz Perlberg Publishing, 2017. *www.doctorgaby.com*

 Do not use without consulting a health practitioner. The elimination diet described below is a modification of a diet recommended by William Crook, M.D., a pioneer in the evaluation and management of hidden food allergy. The purpose of this diet is to identify hidden food allergens that may be causing some or all of your symptoms. During the elimination period, all common allergens are completely eliminated from the diet for 2-3 weeks. After your symptoms improve, foods are added back one at a time, to determine which foods have been causing symptoms.

Foods You Must Avoid:
DAIRY PRODUCTS: Milk, cheese, butter, yogurt, sour cream, cottage cheese, whey, casein, sodium caseinate, calcium caseinate, and any food containing these.

WHEAT: Most breads, spaghetti, noodles, pasta, most flour, baked goods, durum semolina, farina, and many gravies. Although this diet prohibits wheat, it is not a gluten-free diet. Oats, barley, and rye are allowed.

CORN: Whole corn and foods made with corn (such as corn chips, tortillas, popcorn, and breads and other baked goods that list corn as an ingredient). Also avoid products that contain corn oil, vegetable oil from an unspecified source, corn syrup, corn sweetener, dextrose, and glucose.

EGGS: Whites and yolks, and any products that contain eggs.

CITRUS FRUITS: Oranges, grapefruits, lemons, limes, tangerines, and foods that contain citrus fruits.

COFFEE, TEA, AND ALCOHOL: Avoid both caffeinated and decaffeinated coffee, as well as standard (such as Lipton) tea and decaffeinated tea. Herb teas are allowed, except those that contain citrus.

REFINED SUGARS: Avoid table sugar and any foods that contain it, such as candy, soft drinks, pies, cake, cookies, chocolate, sweetened applesauce, etc. Other names for sugar include sucrose, high-fructose corn syrup, corn syrup, corn sweetener, fructose, cane juice, glucose, dextrose, maltose, maltodextrin, and levulose. These must all be avoided. Some patients (depending on their suspected sensitivity to refined sugar) will be allowed 1-3 teaspoons per day of pure, unprocessed honey, maple syrup, or barley malt syrup. This will be decided on an individual basis. Patients restricted from all sugars should not eat dried fruit. Those who are not restricted from all sugars may eat unsulfured (organically grown) dried fruits sparingly. Because little is known about alternative sweeteners such as stevia, they should not be used during the elimination phase.

Honey, maple syrup, or barley syrup: 1-3 teaspoons per day

Food additives: Avoid artificial colors, flavors, preservatives, texturing agents, artificial sweeteners, etc. Most diet sodas and other dietetic foods contain artificial ingredients and must be avoided. Grapes, prunes, and raisins that are not organically grown may contain sulfites and should be avoided.

Any other food you eat 3 times a week or more: Any food you are now eating 3 times a week or more should be avoided and tested later.

Known allergens: Avoid any food you know you are allergic to, even if it is allowed on this diet.

Tap water (including cooking water): Tap water is eliminated in cases where more extreme sensitivity is suspected. If tap water is not allowed, use spring or distilled water bottled in glass or hard plastic. Water bottled in soft (collapsible) plastic containers tends to leach plastic into the water. Bottles with numbers 3 or 7 are likely to leach phthalates. Choose bottles and containers that are free of bisphenol A (BPA). Some water-filtration systems do not take out all potential allergens. Take your water with you, including to

Read labels: Hidden allergens are frequently found in packaged foods. "Flour" usually means wheat; "vegetable oil" may mean corn oil; and casein and whey are dairy products. Make sure your vitamins are free of wheat, corn, sugar, citrus, yeast, and artificial colorings.

Foods You May Eat:
Cereals:
   Hot: Oatmeal, oat bran, cream of rye, Arrowhead Mills Rice and Shine.

Dry: Barbara's or Erewhon's puffed rice, Barbara's Brown Rice Crisps Cereal. Diluted apple juice with apple slices and nuts go well on cereal. You may use soy milk that has no corn oil or sugar added (such as some Eden Soy and Rice Dream products). Most of these foods are available in health food stores and some grocery stores.

GRAINS AND FLOUR PRODUCTS:

Flours: Soy, rice, potato, buckwheat, and bean flours.

Breads: rice. 100% rye, spelt, or millet bread (as long as they do not contain dairy, eggs, sugar, or wheat).

Cooked whole grains: oats, millet, barley, buckwheat groats (kasha), brown rice, brown rice pasta, rice macaroni, spelt (flour and pasta), amaranth, and quinoa. Other: 100% rice cakes (such as Quaker), rice crackers, rye crackers, Orgran Buckwheat Gluten-free Crispbread, flax crackers (from Foods Alive). Blue Dragon Spring Roll Wrappers. Oriental noodles (such as 100% buckwheat Soba noodles from Eden), and Ka-Me Bean Threads. Most of these products are available at health food stores and can be ordered from any grocery store that carries Arrowhead Mills, Bob's Red Mill, Shilo Farms, or Ancient Harvests.

LEGUMES: Soybeans, tofu, lentils, peas, chickpeas, navy beans, kidney beans, black beans, string beans, and others. Dried beans should be soaked overnight. Pour off the water and rinse before cooking. Canned beans often contain added sugar or other potential allergens. Some cooked beans packaged in glass jars (generally sold at health food stores) contain no sugar. You may also use bean dips (like hummus) that do not contain sugar, lemon, or additives. Canned soups such as split pea, lentil, and turkey/vegetable (without additives) may also be used. Companies that make acceptable products include Amy's, Kettle Cuisine, and Imagine Natural Creations.

VEGETABLES AND FRUITS: Use a wide variety. All vegetables except corn and all fruits except citrus are permitted.

PROTEINS: This includes beef, lamb, pork, chicken, turkey, and fish. Lamb rarely causes allergic reactions, and can be used by most people who have multiple sensitivities. Grain/bean casseroles may be used as an alternative to animal foods (see vegetarian cookbooks for recipes). Shrimp and most canned or packaged shellfish (such as lobster, crab, and oysters) may contain sulfites and should be avoided. Canned tuna, salmon and other canned fish are allowed.

Nuts and seeds: Nuts may be eaten raw or roasted (without sugar). To prevent rancidity, nuts and seeds should be kept in an airtight container in the refrigerator. You may also use nut butters (such as peanut butter, almond butter, cashew butter, walnut butter, sesame butter, hemp seed butter, and sesame tahini). Companies that make acceptable products include Full Circle, Arrowhead Mills, and Natalie's. Nut butters go well on celery sticks and crackers. In recipes, freshly ground flaxseed can be used instead of egg. One tablespoon of ground flaxseed with 1/3 cup of water will bind in recipes as well as one egg, but additional leavening may be needed depending on the recipe.

Oils and fats: Sunflower, safflower, olive, sesame, peanut, flaxseed, canola, and soy oils may be used. Do not use corn oil or "vegetable oil" from an unspecified source (which is usually corn oil). Soy, sunflower, and safflower margarines are acceptable from an allergy standpoint, but most margarines contain *trans* fatty acids (which may promote heart disease) and are therefore not recommended. Vegetable spreads and bean spreads (such as hummus) may be used instead of butter or margarine. Ripe avocado can also be spread on sandwiches in place of mayonnaise.

Snacks: Any permitted food can be eaten as a snack any time of day. Acceptable snacks include Danielle Veggie Chips and Gorge Delight's Just Fruit Bars. Other good snacks include celery, carrot sticks, and other vegetables/ fruit (no citrus); and unsalted fresh nuts and seeds.

Beverages: Acceptable drinks include spring water in glass bottles or hard plastic; herb teas (no lemon or orange); non-citrus fruit juices without sugar or additives (dilute 50:50 with water); and soy or rice milk without corn oil (such as Eden Soy Plain or Rice Dream Original). Caffix, Inka, and Kafree Roma may be used as coffee substitutes. Tap water contains chlorine, fluoride, and other potentially allergenic chemicals. In some cases, spring water in glass or hard-plastic bottles is the only water allowed. This would include water used for cooking. If tap water is eliminated, it should be reintroduced as if it were a test food. Restrictions on the type of water permitted will be made on a case-by-case basis.

THICKENERS: Rice, oat, millet, barley, soy, or amaranth flours; arrowroot powder; agar flakes; and kudzu powder may be used as thickeners.

SPICES AND CONDIMENTS: Acceptable items include salt (in moderation), pepper, herbal spices (without preservatives, citrus, or sugar), garlic, ginger, onions, catsup and mustard without sugar (such as catsup from Muir Glen and mustard from Full Circle), Bragg Liquid Aminos (as a replacement for soy sauces that contain wheat or additives), and Vitamin C crystals in water (as a substitute for lemon juice).

MISCELLANEOUS FOODS: Sugar-free spaghetti sauce (such as Amy's) and fruit jellies without sugar or citrus (such as Suzanne's fruit spreads).

General Suggestions:

Do NOT RESTRICT CALORIES: Start with a good breakfast, eat frequently throughout the day, and consume at least 4 glasses of water per day. If you do not eat enough, you may experience symptoms of low blood sugar, such as fatigue, irritability, headache, and rapid weight loss. Eat a wide variety of foods. Do not rely on just a few foods, because you may become allergic to foods you eat every day. To ensure adequate fiber intake, eat beans, permitted whole grains, whole fruits and vegetables, homemade vegetable soup, nuts, and seeds. Be sure to chew thoroughly, in order to enhance digestion.

PLAN MEALS: Plan your meals for the entire week. Take some time before starting the diet, in order to develop meal plans and stock the kitchen with adequate amounts of permitted foods. For ideas, look through cookbooks that specialize in hypoallergenic diets. Most meals can be modified easily to meet the requirements of the diet, without changing the meal plan for the rest of your family. When you go to the health food store, ask for assistance in locating appropriate breads, crackers, cereals, soups, etc. Some people find it useful to prepare additional foods on the weekend, which helps to cut down on thinking and preparation time during the week. If you need further assistance or ideas, contact your doctor or health practitioner.

DINING OUT: Do not hesitate to ask questions or make requests. For example, you could ask for fish topped with slivered almonds, cooked without added seasoning, butter or lemon. Get baked potato with a slice of onion on top. Order steak or lamb chops with fresh vegetables, also prepared without added seasonings (with the exception of garlic and plain herbs). Make sure the salad bar does not use sulfites as preservative, and bring your own dressing (oil and cider vinegar with chopped nuts/seeds and fresh herbs). Carry pure water, snacks, seasonings, etc., wherever you go, to supplement your meals or to have something on hand if you get hungry.

WITHDRAWAL SYMPTOMS: About 1 in 4 patients develop mild "withdrawal" symptoms within a few days after starting the diet. Withdrawal symptoms may include fatigue, irritability, headaches, malaise, or increased hunger. These symptoms generally disappear within 2-5 days and are usually followed by an improvement to your original symptoms. If withdrawal symptoms are too uncomfortable, take buffered vitamin C (sodium ascorbate or calcium ascorbate) at a dose of 1,000 mg in tablet/capsule form or ¼ teaspoon of the crystals, up to 4 times per day. Your doctor may also prescribe alkali salts (a mixture of sodium bicarbonate and potassium bicarbonate, taken as needed at a dose of ¼ to ½ teaspoon dissolved in 6-8 ounces of water up to 3-4 times per day). In most cases, withdrawal symptoms are not severe and do not require treatment. When starting the elimination diet, it is best to discontinue all of the foods abruptly ("cold turkey"), rather than easing into the diet slowly.

Testing Individual Foods:
It usually takes 2-3 weeks for symptoms to improve enough to allow you to retest foods. However, you may begin retesting sooner if you have been feeling a lot better for at least 5 days and have been on the diet for at least 10 days. If you have been on the diet for 4 weeks and feel no better, contact your doctor or health practitioner for further instructions. Most patients do improve. Some feel so much better on the diet that they decide not to test the foods. This could be a mistake. If you wait too long to retest, your allergies may "settle down" and you will not be able to provoke symptoms of food testing. As a result, you will not know which foods you are allergic to. If reintroducing certain foods causes a recurrence of symptoms, you are probably allergic to those foods.

FOOD SOURCES FOR TESTING: Test pure sources of the various foods. For example, do not use pizza to test cheese, because pizza also contains wheat and possibly corn oil. Do not use bread to test wheat, because bread often contains other potential allergens. It is best to use organic foods for testing, so as not to risk interference from pesticides, hormones, or other additives that may be present in some foods.

TESTING PROCEDURE: Test one new food each day. If your main symptom is arthritic pain, test one new food every other day. Allergic reactions to test foods usually occur within 10 minutes to 12 hours after ingestion. However, joint pains may be delayed by as much as 48 hours. Eat a relatively large amount of each test food. For example, on the day you test milk, consume a large glass at breakfast, along with any of the other foods on the "permitted" list. If, after one serving, your original symptoms come back, or if you develop a headache, bloating, nausea, dizziness, or fatigue, do not eat that food again and place it on your "allergic" list. If no symptoms occur, eat the food again for lunch and dinner and watch for reactions. Even if the food is well tolerated, do not add it back into your diet until you have finished testing all of the foods. If you do experience a reaction, wait until your symptoms have improved before testing the next food. In some instances, it may not be clear whether the symptoms you are experiencing are due to the most recently eaten food or to a delayed reaction to a previously eaten food. If you are uncertain whether you have reacted to a particular food, remove it from your diet and retest it 4-5 days later. You do not have to test foods you never eat. Do not test foods you already know cause symptoms.

Foods may be tested in any order. Begin testing on a day you are feeling well. Keep a daily journal that records individual food challenges and symptoms.

DAIRY TESTS: Test milk and cheese on separate days. You may wish to test several cheeses on different days, since some people are allergic to certain cheeses but not to others. It is usually not necessary to test yogurt, cottage cheese, or butter separately.

WHEAT TEST: Use Wheatena (with no milk or sugar) or another pure wheat cereal. You may add soy or rice milk.

CORN TEST: Use fresh ears of corn or frozen corn (without sauces or preservatives).

Egg test: Test the whites and yolks on separate days, using hard-boiled eggs.

Citrus test: Test oranges, grapefruits, lemons, and limes individually on separate days. The lemon and lime can be squeezed into water. For oranges and grapefruits, use whole, fresh fruit.

Tap water and frequently eaten foods: Test tap water, if you have eliminated it. Also, test the foods you have eliminated because they were being eaten frequently.

Optional Tests:

If any of the items below are not now a part of your diet, or if you are committed to eliminating them from your diet, there is no need to test them. However, if you have been consuming any of these items regularly, it is a good idea to test them and find out how they affect you. Reactions to these foods and beverages may be severe in some cases. They should be tested only on days that you can afford to feel bad.

Coffee and tea: Test on separate days. Do not add milk, non dairy creamer, or sugar, but an acceptable soy or rice milk may be added. If you use decaffeinated coffee, test it separately. Coffee, tea, decaffeinated coffee, and decaffeinated tea are separate tests.

Sugar: Put 4 teaspoons of cane sugar in a drink or on cereal, or mix it with another food.

Chocolate: Use 1-2 tablespoons of pure baker's chocolate or Hershey's cocoa powder.

Food additives: Buy a set of McCormick or French's food dyes and colors. Put ½ teaspoon of each color in a glass. Add one teaspoon of the mixture to a glass of water and drink. If you wish, you may test each color separately.

Alcohol: Beer, wine, and hard liquor may require testing on different days, since the reactions to each may be different. Have 2 drinks per test day, but only if you can afford not to feel well that day and possibly the next day.

Suggestions for Self-Help:
Rotation diet: If you have an allergic constitution and eat the same foods every day, you may eventually become allergic to those foods. After you have discovered which foods you can eat safely, make an attempt to rotate your diet. A 4-day schedule is necessary for some highly allergic people, but most people can tolerate foods more frequently than every 4 days. You may eventually be able to tolerate allergenic foods, after you have avoided them for 6-12 months. However, if you continue to eat these foods more frequently than every fourth day, the allergy may return.

Consume a wide variety of foods, not just a few favorites. If you are rotating foods, be sure to avoid all forms of the food when you are on an "off" day. For example, if you are rotating corn, avoid corn chips, corn oil, corn sweeteners, etc., except on the days you are eating corn and corn products. It is not necessary to do strict food rotation during the elimination and retesting periods.

Watch for other allergic reactions: If you have an allergic constitution, you may be allergic to foods other than those you have eliminated and tested on this diet. Pay attention to what you are eating, and review recent meals if you develop symptoms. You can then eliminate that food for 2 weeks and test it again, to see if it triggers the same symptoms.

Reference: Crook, W. *Tracking Down Hidden Food Allergy*, Jackson, TN: Professional Books, 1980.

Note: Health-food stores or libraries frequently carry a wide variety of books on self-help literature on the subject of food preparation for allergic people.

Lab Tests
Laboratories that test for food allergies:

Elisa Act Biotechnologies
109 Carpenter Drive
Suite 100
Sterling, VA 20164
Phone: 1-800-553-5472
E-mail: *clientservices@Elisaact.com*
Website: *www.elisaact.com*

Genova Diagnostics
63 Zukkucia Street
Asheville, NC 28801
Phone: 1-800-522-4762
Website: *www.gdx.net*

US BioTek Laboratories
16020 Linden Ave N.
Shoreline, WA 98133-5672
Phone: 1-877-318-8728
E-mail: *cservice@usbiotek.com*
Website: *www.usbiotek.com*

Books

William Crook, M.D. *Tracking the Hidden Food Allergy.* Jackson, TN: Professional Books, 1980.

William Davis, M.D. *Wheatbelly: Lose the Wheat, Lose the Weight, and Find Your Path Back to Health.* New York: Rodale, 2011.

_____. *The Wheatbelly Cookbook.* New York: Rodale, 2013.

Alan R. Gaby, M.D. *Nutritional Medicine.* 2nd Edition. Concord, NH: Fritz Perlberg Publishing, 2017.

Cybele Pascal. *The Whole Foods Allergy Cookbook.* Ridgefield, CT: Vital Health Publishing, 2006.

CHAPTER THREE—NUTRITION: FINDING YOUR *NOURISHING* RHYTHM

Food Log

A ONE WEEK FOOD DIARY CHART *(LOG IN FOODS EATEN AND TIMES. NOTES THE SYMPTOMS YOU HAVE AND WHAT TIMES AS WELL)*							
	DAY 1	DAY 2	DAY 3	DAY 4	DAY 5	DAY 6	DAY 7
MORNING FOODS							
MORNING SYMPTOMS							
AFTERNOON FOODS							
AFTERNOON SYMPTOMS							
EVENING FOODS							
EVENING SYMPTOMS							

Energy Balls Recipe

(Makes about 3 dozen)

¼ cup sesame seeds
¼ cup sunflower seeds
½ cup raisins
½ cup dried figs
½ cup peanut butter, almond butter, or tahini
½ cup coconut oil
1 tsp vanilla
cinnamon to taste

Place sesame seeds, sunflower seeds, raisins and figs in a food processor with a metal blade. Chop until everything is ground together. Add nut or seed butter and mix until combined. Roll mixture into balls, or press into an 8-inch round cake pan and cut into 1-inch squares. Keep refrigerated.

Note: Nuts can be substituted for seeds. Other dried fruit, such as mango and apricot, can be substituted for raisins and figs. Additional protein can be added with ¼ cup spirulina.

Variation: Coconut Energy Bars: Add ½ cup unsweetened coconut to mixture. Add a little coconut milk, if necessary, to help balls hold together.

A Shopper's Guide to Pesticides in Produce

Highest in Pesticides

Apples	Peaches
Bell Peppers	Pears
Celery	Potatoes
Cherries	Red Raspberries
Grapes (imported)	Spinach
Nectarines	Strawberries

Lowest in Pesticides

Asparagus	Kiwi
Avocados	Mangos
Bananas	Onions
Broccoli	Papaya
Cauliflower	Pineapple
Corn (sweet)	Peas (sweet)

Lab Tests

Here are some labs that test for vitamin deficiencies:

Genova Diagnostics
63 Zukkucia Street
Asheville, NC 28801
Phone: 1-800-522-4762
Website: *www.gdx.net*

Great Plains Laboratory, Inc.
11813 West 77th Street
Lenexa, KS 66214
Phone: 1-800-288-0383
E-mail: *customerservice@gpl4u.com*
Website: *www.greatplainslaboratory.com*

SpectraCell Laboratories
10401 Town Park Drive
Houston, TX 77072
Phone: 1-800-227-5227
E-mail: *spec1@spectracell.com*
Website: *www.spectracell.com*

Books

Sally Fallon, with Mary Enig, Ph.D. *Nourishing Traditions.* Washington, DC: New Trends Publishing, 1999.

Sandor Ellix Katz. *Wild Fermentation.* White River Junction, VT: Chelsea Green Publishing Company, 2003.

Weston A. Price, D.D.S. *Nutrition and Physical Degeneration.* La Mesa, CA: The Price-Pottenger Nutrition Foundation, 1939.

Lorna J. Sass. *Recipes from an Ecological Kitchen.* New York: William Morrow & Co., 1992.

Nina Teicholz. *The Big Fat Surprise.* New York: Simon & Schuster, 2014.

Vitamin Companies (a partial list)
Thorne, Perque, Standard Process, Biotics.

CHAPTER FIVE—THE MIND-BODY CONNECTION

Bach Flower Remedies

Following is the list of the Bach Flowers, along with the particular thought pattern for which each plant is a remedy. One chooses the remedies that reflect the negative thought patterns one is experiencing. If the treatment is successful, the thought patterns stop repeating. The remedies can be taken as 4 drops on the tongue as often as needed, or by adding 4 drops to a glass of water.

AGRIMONY	Attempts to conceal torturing thoughts and inner restlessness behind a façade of cheerfulness and freedom from care.
ASPEN	Inexplicable vague fears, apprehensions, a secret fear of some impending evil.

BEECH	Critical attitude, arrogance, intolerance, criticizing without any understanding of the views and situation of others.
CENTAURY	Weak-willed overreaction to the wishes of others; good-natured, easily exploited, can't say no.
CERATO	Doubting of own judgment, and having the need to seek the confirmation of others.
CHESTNUT BUD	Repeating the same faults over and over again, due to lack of learning from experience.
CHICORY	Possessive, excessively interfering, manipulating in the affairs of others, being absorbed in self-pity support from others.
CLEMATIS	Daydreaming, inattentiveness, and paying little attention to the goings-on around oneself.
ELM	Overwhelmed by responsibility.
GENTIAN	Skeptical, doubting, pessimistic, and easily discouraged.
GORSE	Long-term suffering from chronic disease that produces negative expectations. The attitude reinforces disease.
HEATHER	Always needs an audience; irresistible urge to off-load everything that happens to them.
HOLLY	Hatred, envy, jealousy, and suspicion.
HONEYSUCKLE	Need to cling to the past, being overly nostalgic or homesick.
HORNBEAM	Great weariness and exhaustion, largely in the mind.
IMPATIENS	Impatience, intolerance, irritability.
LARCH	Lack of self-confidence, sense of inferiority, and fear of failure.
MIMULUS	Fear of known things, shyness and timidity.
MUSTARD	"Dark cloud" that descends, making one saddened and low for no known reason.

OAK	Strength and courage with a need to fight against great odds, and never knowing when to let go of the fight.
OLIVE	Exhaustion, drained energy.
PINE	Guilt complex—blaming self, even for mistakes of others.
RED CHESTNUT	Excessive concern and worry over others.
ROCK ROSE	Suddenly alarmed, panicky, experiencing terror or fright.
ROCK WATER	The pleasures of life are suffocated under self-imposed disciplines.
SCLERANTHUS	Indecisive, erratic, lacking inner balance; fluctuating mood.
SWEET CHESTNUT	Hopeless despair of those who feel they have reached the limit of their endurance.
VERVAIN	Overly enthusiastic; highly-strung and even fanatical.
VINE	Dominating, inflexible, striving for power.
WALNUT	Difficulties of adjusting in transition periods of life.
WATER VIOLET	"Loners," need of being alone, little emotional involvement.
WHITE CHESTNUT	Unwanted thoughts keep going around in one's head; mental arguments and dialogues.
WILD OAT	Dissatisfaction because one's mission in life is not found.
WILD ROSE	Resignation; lack of interest and ambition; apathy.
WILLOW	Unspoken resentment, bitterness, "poor me" or "victim of fate" attitude.
RESCUE REMEDY	Trauma, numbness, terror, panic, irritability, tension and fear.

Essential Oils

There are many companies providing these oils, which are available through both retail and multilevel marketing. The ones I have used the most are:

Aroma Medica, by Dr. Geraldine DePaula
www.aromamedica.com

Mikael Zayat's company:
Zayat Aroma
1339 Shefford, Bromont, Qc, Canada J2L1C9
E-mail: *info@zayataroma.com*
Phone: 1-855-534-1671
Fax: 1-855-318-6124

Books

James Hollis, Ph.D. *Swamplands of the Soul: New Life in Dismal Places.* Toronto, Canada: Inner City Books, 1996.

Daniel Keown, M.B. Ch.B., M.C.E.M., Lic. Ac. *The Spark in the Machine.* London: Singing Dragon, 2014.

James L. Oschman. *Energy Medicine, The Scientific Basis.* London: Churchill Livingstone, 2000.

Candace Pert, Ph.D. *Molecules of Emotion.* New York: Simon & Schuster, 1997.

Julia Ross, M.A. *The Mood Cure.* London: Penguin Books, 2004

Chapter Six—Puberty and Beyond

Red Tent Groups

For more information on Red Tent activities, see:
www.redtenttemplemovement.com

Lab Tests

Here are some labs that test for hormones:

Doctor's Data, Inc.
3755 Illinois Avenue
St. Charles, IL 60174-2420

Phone: 1-800-323-2784
E-mail: *info@doctorsdata.com*
Website: *www.doctorsdata.com*

Genova Diagnostics
63 Zukkucia Street
Asheville, NC 28801
Phone: 1-800-522-4762
Website: *www.gdx.net*

US BioTek Laboratories
16020 Linden Ave N.
Shoreline, WA 98133-5672
Phone: 1-877-318-8728
E-mail: *cservice@usbiotek.com*
Website: *www.usbiotek.com*

Books

General

Boston Women's Health Collective. *Our Bodies Ourselves.* New York: Simon and Schuster, 1971

Christiane Northrop, M.D. *Women's Bodies, Women's Wisdom.* New York: Bantam Books, 1994.

Adolescence

Mahdi / Christopher/Meade, editors. *Crossroads: The Quest for Contemporary Rites of Passage.* Chicago: Open Court Publishing, 1996.

Mary Pipher, Ph.D. *Reviving Ophelia: Saving the Selves of Adolescent Girls.* New York: Penguin, 1994.

Marion Woodman. *Addiction to Perfection.* New York: Ballantine Books, 1996.

Pregnancy and Childbirth

Ina May Gaskin. *Guide to Childbirth.* New York: Bantam Dell / Random House, 2003.

Erna Wright. *The New Childbirth.* London: The Book Service Ltd., 1964.

CHAPTER SEVEN—MENOPAUSE

Bone Broth Recipe

Ingredients

About 4 pounds beef marrow and knuckle bones

1 calf's foot, cut into pieces (optional)

3 pounds meaty rib or neck bones

4 or more quarts cold filtered water

½ cup vinegar

3 onions, coarsely chopped

3 carrots, coarsely chopped

3 celery stalks, coarsely chopped

Several sprigs of fresh thyme, tied together

1 teaspoon dried green peppercorns, crushed

1 bunch parsley

Directions

Good beef stock must be made with several sorts of bones: knuckle bones and feet impart large quantities of particular nutrients of bone marrows; and meaty rib or neck bones add color and flavor.

Place the knuckle and marrow bones and optional calf's foot in a very large pot with vinegar, and cover with water. Let stand for one hour. Meanwhile, place the meaty bones in a roasting pan and brown at 350 degrees in the oven. When well browned, add to the pot along with the vegetables. Pour the fat out of the roasting pan, add cold water to the pan, set over a high flame, and bring to a boil, stirring with a wooden spoon to loosen up coagulated juices. Add this liquid to the pot. Add additional water, if necessary, to cover the bones; but the liquid should come no higher than within an inch of the rim of the pot, as the volume expands slightly during cooking. Bring to a boil. A large amount of scum will come to the top, and it is important to remove this with a spoon. After you have skimmed, reduce heat and add the thyme and crushed peppercorns.

Simmer stock for at least 12 and as long as 72 hours. Just before finishing, add the parsley and simmer for another 10 minutes.

You will now have a pot of rather repulsive-looking brown liquid containing globs of gelatinous and fatty material. It doesn't even smell particularly good. But don't despair. After straining, you will have a delicious and nourishing clear broth that forms that basis for many other recipes.

Remove bones with tongs or a slotted spoon. Strain the stock into a large bowl. Let cool in the refrigerator and remove the congealed fat that rises to the top. Transfer to smaller containers and to the freezer for long-term storage.

Variation: Lamb Stock: Use *lamb bones,* especially lamb neck bones and riblets. This makes a delicious stock.

Variation: Venison Stock: Use *venison meat and bones.* Be sure to use the feet of the deer and a section of antler, if possible.

Books

Alan Gaby, M.D. *Preventing and Reversing Osteoporosis.* Rocklin, CA.: Prima Publishing, 1994.

John Lee, M.D., and Virginia Hopkins. *What Your Doctor May Not Tell You About Menopause.* New York: Warner Books, 1996.

Christiane Northrup, M.D. *The Wisdom of Menopause.* New York: Bantam Books, 2001.

CHAPTER EIGHT—SEXUALITY

Books

Alison A. Armstrong. *Keys to the Kingdom.* Sherman Oaks, CA: PAX Programs, 2003.

_____. *The Queen's Code.* Sherman Oaks, CA: PAX Programs, 2013.

Betty Dodson. *Sex for One.* New York: Three Rivers Press, 1996.

Eugene Shippen, M.D. *The Testosterone Syndrome.* New York: M. Evans and Company, 1998.

Suzanne Somers. *The Sexy Years: Discover the Hormone Connection.* New York: Harmony Books, Random House, *2003.*

Sheri Winston, CNM, RN, BSN. *Women's Anatomy of Arousal: Secret Maps to Buried Treasure.* New York: Mango Garden Press, 2010.

Naomi Wolf. *Vagina: A New Biography.* London: Little, Brown, 2012.

CHAPTER NINE—FATIGUE AND RECOVERY

Candida Quiz

From Dr. William Crook's book, *The Yeast Connection Handbook.*

Are Your Health Problems Yeast Connected?

If your answer is "yes" to any question, circle the number in the right hand column. When you've completed the questionnaire, add up the points you've circled. Your score will help you determine the possibility (or probability) that your health problems are yeast connected.

YES SCORE

Have you taken repeated or prolonged courses of antibacterial drugs?	4
Have you been bothered by recurrent vaginal, prostate, or urinary infections?	3
Do you feel "sick all over," yet the cause hasn't been found?	2
Are you bothered by hormone disturbances, including PMS, menstrual irregularities, sexual dysfunction, sugar craving, low body temperature, or fatigue?	2
Are you unusually sensitive to tobacco smoke, perfumes, colognes, and other chemical odors?	2
Are you bothered by memory or concentration problems? Do you sometimes feel "spaced out"?	2
Have you taken prolonged courses of prednisone or other steroids; or have you taken "the pill" for more than 3 years?	2
Do some foods disagree with you or trigger your symptoms?	1
Do you suffer with constipation, diarrhea, bloating, or abdominal pain?	1
Does your skin itch, tingle or burn; or is it unusually dry; or are you bothered by rashes?	1

Scoring for women: If your score is 9 or more, your health problems are probably yeast connected. If your score is 12 or more, your health problems are almost certainly yeast connected.

Scoring for men: If your score is 7 or more, your health problems are probably yeast connected. If you score is 10 or more, your health problems are almost certainly yeast connected.

Books

Broda O. Barnes, M.D., and Lawrence Galton. *Hypothyroidism: The Unsuspected Illness.*
New York: Harper & Row, 1976.

William G. Crook, M.D. *The Yeast Connection Handbook: How Yeasts Can Make You Feel "Sick All Over" and the Steps You Need to Take to Regain Your Health.* Jackson, TN: Professional Books, Inc., 1995.

Jacob Teitelbaum, M.D. *From Fatigued to Fantastic.* London: Penguin Books, 2007.

_____. *The Fatigue and Fibromyalgia Solution.* London: Penguin Books, 2013.

⌒♪

CHAPTER TEN—OPTIMAL AGEING: THE CROWN OF LIFE

Books

Margaret Atwood. *The Blind Assassin: A Novel.* Toronto: Random House/Anchor, 2001.

Nora Ephron. *I Remember Nothing: And Other Reflections.* New York: Knopf Doubleday Publishing Group, 2010.

Atul Gawande, M.D. *Being Mortal: Medicine and What Matters in the End.* New York: Metropolitan Books, 2014.

James Hollis, Ph.D. *Finding Meaning in the Second Half of Life: How to Finally, Really Grow Up.* London: Gotham Books, 2005.

Elizabeth Kubler-Ross, M.D. *Remember the Secret.* New York: Tricycle Press, 1998.

Kathryn Mannix. *With the End in Mind: How to Live and Die Well.* Great Britain: William Collins, 2017.

Jessye Norman. *Stand Up Straight and Sing!* New York: Houghton Mifflin Harcourt, 2014.

Sherwin B. Nuland. *How We Die.* New York: Vintage Books, 1993.

Articles

Richard Horton, *The Lancet*, Vol. 394 (October 12, 2019).

~~~

EPILOGUE

American Board of Integrative and Holistic Medicine
www.aihm.org
info@aihm.org

Institute for Functional Medicine
www.ifm.org

American Association of Naturopathic Physicians
www.naturopathic.org

American Naturopathic Association
www.naturopathic.org

American Naturopathic Medical Association
www.anma.org

Association of Accredited Naturopathic Medical Colleges
https://aanmc.org

National Ayurvedic Medical Association
www.ayurvedanama.org

National Certification Commission for Acupuncture and Oriental Medicine
www.nccaom.org

Glossary

Antibodies:

    Antithyroglobulin antibodies — another antibody that can block the effectiveness of thyroid hormone.

    TPO Antibodies — Thyroid Peroxidase antibodies, which can block the availability of thyroid hormone.

CBC — Complete Blood Count. It should also include a differential that delineates how many of each different kind of blood cells are present.

CBT — Cognitive-behavioral therapy (CBT) is a psycho-social intervention that is the most widely used evidence-based practice for improving mental health. Guided by empirical research, CBT focuses on the development of personal coping strategies that target solving current problems and changing unhelpful patterns in cognitions (e.g. thoughts, beliefs, and attitudes), behaviors, and emotional regulation.

    According to *Psychology Today* (the website), cognitive behavioral therapy (CBT) is a short-term form of psychotherapy directed at present-time issues and based on the idea that the way an individual thinks and feels affects the way he or she behaves. The focus is on problem solving, and the goal is to change clients' thought patterns in order to change their responses to difficult situations. A CBT approach can be applied to a wide range of mental health issues and conditions. Further information can be found on their website: *https://www.psychologytoday.com/therapy-types/cognitive-behavioral-therapy-0*

DHEA — dehydroepiandrosterone.

Dyslipidemia — a term used to describe elevated cholesterol levels.

Ferritin — a storage form of iron.

Hashimoto's hypothyroid — a particular subset of hypothyroid conditions where there are abnormally high levels of thyroid antibodies. The antibodies interfere with thyroid function.

MCV (Mean Corpuscular Volume) — Lack of either Vitamin B12 or folate or both can result in raising the MCV, which means that the size of the red blood cells, or corpuscles, are larger than the normal range. Even if the MCV is in the higher end of the normal range, this can indicate that some B12 or folate insufficiency is present.

mIU/L — milli International Units per Liter of blood.

Pg/mL — picograms per milliliter.

RDW — red blood cell distribution width. If anemia is observed, RDW test results are often used together with mean corpuscular volume (MCV) results to determine the possible causes of the anemia and how the body is responding.

T3 and T4:

> **T4** — the hormone produced by the thyroid gland.

> **T3** — the hormone converted from T4 that is produced in the body, mainly in the liver.

> **Free T4 and Free T3** — the amounts of active thyroid hormone that are *actually available* to bind with thyroid receptor sites.

> **Reverse T3** — this is an *inactive* form of T3.

TIBC — Total iron binding capacity. TIBC is a blood test to see if you have too much or too little iron in the blood. Iron moves through the blood attached to a protein called transferrin. The TIBC test helps your doctor know how much iron is attached to transferrin.

USP — a standardized prescription dose monitored by the FDA.

About the Author

Marianne Rothschild, M.D., is a family physician who has practiced holistic medicine for over forty years, thirty of which she has been a physician. She blends many traditions of healing in her work, including herbs, nutrition, lifestyle counseling, homeopathy, flower essences, and aromatherapy, in addition to conventional Western medicine.

She received her medical degree from the Medical College of Pennsylvania in 1990 with honors in emergency medicine and community and preventive medicine. She completed her family practice residency at Chestnut Hill Hospital in Philadelphia.

After moving to Maryland, Dr. Rothschild worked with the Johns Hopkins Medical Services Corporation before establishing her own practice. She has grown children, many grandchildren, and currently has a private practice in Maryland. More information can be found on her website: *www.dancingwiththerhythmsoflife.com* and *www.mariannerothschildmd.com*.

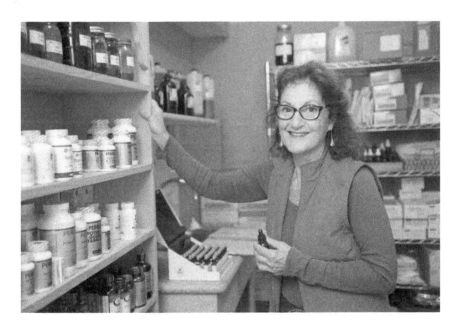

CPSIA information can be obtained
at www.ICGtesting.com
Printed in the USA
JSHW030212040822
28752JS00001B/3